S. HRG. 109–376

FIELD HEARING ON THE STATE OF VA CARE IN HAWAII: PART I

HEARING

BEFORE THE

COMMITTEE ON VETERANS' AFFAIRS
UNITED STATES SENATE

ONE HUNDRED NINTH CONGRESS

SECOND SESSION

JANUARY 10, 2006

Printed for the use of the Committee on Veterans' Affairs

Available via the World Wide Web: http://www.access.gpo.gov/congress/senate

U.S. GOVERNMENT PRINTING OFFICE

27-350 PDF   WASHINGTON : 2006

CONTENTS

JANUARY 10, 2006

SENATORS

WITNESSES

APPENDIX 1

APPENDIX 2

JANUARY 9, 2006—HAWAII HEARING, KAUI

"

FIELD HEARING ON THE STATE OF VA CARE IN HAWAII

TUESDAY, JANUARY 10, 2006

U.S. SENATE,
COMMITTEE ON VETERANS' AFFAIRS,
Washington, DC.

The Committee met, pursuant to notice, at 10:10 a.m., in the J. Walter Cameron Center Auditorium, 95 Mahalani Street, Kahului, Hawaii, Hon. Larry Craig (Chairman of the Committee) presiding.

Present: Senators Craig and Akaka.

OPENING STATEMENT OF HON. LARRY CRAIG, U.S. SENATOR FROM IDAHO

Chairman CRAIG. Good morning, ladies and gentlemen.

AUDIENCE MEMBERS. Good morning. Aloha.

Chairman CRAIG. Aloha. Thank you very much. It is a tremendous pleasure of mine to bring the Senate Committee on Veterans' Affairs to Maui, and to have an opportunity to visit with many of you today on issues that affect all veterans. I say that to receive testimony on the state of VA care here in Hawaii and on the neighboring islands of this great State is not only an opportunity for me, but an honor.

As some of you may know, we held hearings yesterday on the island of—I always work on these names—Kauai——

Senator AKAKA. Kauai.

Chairman CRAIG. Danny corrects me—that focused on VA's long-term care programs nationally and here in Hawaii.

What a beautiful setting for a hearing, I said as we landed this morning, and there was a rainbow. Is there always a rainbow in Hawaii? I suspect so. Well, I'll tell you. It lifts the spirit and the attitude. Rarely do you see a rainbow in Washington, DC.

Yesterday after the hearing, we flew back to Oahu and spent the afternoon out at the National Memorial Cemetery of the Pacific. What a phenomenal and humbling experience. And, of course, at Pearl Harbor. Spent some time, once again, looking down into the waters of the Arizona.

I was truly awestruck when I saw these sights and the events that drew our great country into World War II. Of course, I was a very small child at that time. In fact, my parents would suggest I hadn't even been thought of yet. But I must tell you that it is that and your history, the history of the people of this great State, that is so long and proud in their defense of America's freedoms that you have always met the challenge for. Of course, we, both

"

Danny and I, in understanding that, recognize our jobs as honoring America's heroes.

I am pleased to be here with my friend, and I say that most sincerely, Senator Danny Akaka. Senator Akaka and I came to Congress at about the same time. We served in the House together for a decade. We came to the Senate in 1990. Now we find ourselves as the senior Members of the Veterans' Affairs Committee.

Early on in that relationship, he invited me to Hawaii, and of course, I invited him to Idaho. For some strange reason, he wanted me to come here in August. I said, you know, we've got these roles reversed. You come to Idaho in August. I'll come to Hawaii in January or February. It snowed in Idaho yesterday, and the skiing there is excellent at this moment. And it's obvious why we're here now, and not there. But Danny has been to my beautiful State before, and we hope to get him out there again.

Senator Akaka has been vocal in his belief that Hawaii has a unique geographic issue that other Members of Congress must experience firsthand to understand this great State. I agree with my colleague that there is no substitute for personal and on-the-ground experience. That's why I'm here at Danny's request. And that's why we're spending the time that we are with the four hearings. This is the second of four scheduled across the State.

For those in the audience who don't know much about Idaho, Idaho and Hawaii are very similar in the sense of geography and distance—difficulty of movement. You may have water; we have high mountains. And at times, during this time of the year in Idaho, it can be very, very difficult to move from one community to the other.

Traveling the length of my State is a 500-mile journey. Traveling the width of my State at one point is a near 500-mile journey. So, there are great commonalities between our States as it relates to the geographic issues. And therefore, how do we service and how do we provide service to men and women who choose to live, as they have the right to, in small rural communities across our States?

That is an issue here. It is an issue in Idaho. It's why we're here to see how we might improve those services, or offer different types of services that meet certainly the requirements of all of you and all of your needs. Mental health treatment is often very difficult to come by, and extensive travel, often measured in hundreds of miles, can be required to receive complex surgical care.

I mention this because of our uniqueness as States and our relationship as friends. I say to all of you that if all of our country's Senators were as kind, as hardworking, and as generous as Danny Akaka, the Senate would be an even better place to work. I trust that you feel privileged to have him serving you in the U.S. Senate because I feel privileged to view him as one of my friends.

So I will turn to Danny now for his opening comments, and then he's going to introduce the first panel. We have two panels this morning. Our time is limited because we want to get on and visit a CBOC and the Vets Center and get out on the ground, after testimony and after listening to your concerns and responding to some of the questions that we may have coming out of our panels' testimony.

So with that, let me turn the microphone to Senator Akaka.
Danny.
[Applause.]

OPENING STATEMENT OF HON. DANIEL K. AKAKA, U.S. SENATOR FROM HAWAII

Senator AKAKA. Mahalo. Mahalo nui loa to all of you. And I want to say an extra mahalo nui loa to the Chairman for coming here to Hawaii to all these hearings. And I want to thank the Chairman for his generous remarks this morning.

I want to tell you that as he mentioned, we've worked together for many years. Larry Craig was a great Congressmen and is a great Senator. He's inching up in leadership in the Senate. So don't be surprised if you see Larry Craig from Idaho as one of the leaders of the U.S. Senate one of these days.

And I really treasure his friendship. I must tell you that since he took over and we became leaders of the Veterans' Committee, that Committee is moving.

And I want to tell you that we share many of the same ideas. There's no question that we want to do the best we can to help the veterans. I think you know that there are limits, but we want to do the best we can within the limits to give all the services we can to the veterans of our country.

In Hawaii, we have, as the Chairman mentioned, unique issues because of geography and because of our culture. Other States have similar problems. This hearing will really help the Committee to try to do a job that's great.

We have the top people here from VA, nationally, as well as Statewide, and region-wide, too, here with us to testify. But we are all here to try to see what we can do to help the veterans. That's our effort here.

So I'm so glad. I also want you to know that this is the first hearing where the Chairman of the Committee has traveled to Hawaii in the history of our country.

[Applause.]

Senator AKAKA. Thanks to the Chairman and our staffs, who worked so hard to bring this about. I want to tell you that normally the Committee doesn't leave Washington, DC. for hearings. We have hearings in Washington. So this is very rare. But we are very privileged to have the Committee out here. For me, too, I mean, it's kind of a thrill to be able to bring the Committee out here to Hawaii.

As I said, the Chairman has really had a busy schedule, at home and in Washington. But I was so glad to have him, as he said, suggest it: Hey, if not August, what about January? Oh, that's all right with me. You know, whenever it is. And it worked out beautifully because I feel great being home in Hawaii whenever I can come home. And thanks to the Chairman for all of this. And we are privileged and honored that all of you have come to testify here and to listen to the testimony about the needs of Hawaii's veterans.

You know, I want to mention—I'm taking long—but I want to mention about what the Chairman said about the rainbow. You know, the rainbow is very symbolic and important to Hawaii. I come from a place on Oahu, and we always have rainbows. I remember my mom, my father and mother, would always tell me, "The rainbow is here."

And it's a kind of symbol that is beautiful. It's spiritual in a way because you can't touch it. It's there. It represents hope. It's beautiful because it represents all the colors. It's good for Hawaii because Hawaii is diverse. It has many, many ethnic groups, and each ethnic group is in that rainbow. The way I like to put it is that, whatever ethnic person you are, it's good to know your tradition. When you do that, your color is bright. But your color is better when it's side by side with other colors.

That's why we're here. You know, we harmonize. We work together. And that's a rainbow. There's a song that I call the rainbow song, but it's really beautiful and it has lots of meaning. I'm so glad the Chairman mentioned the rainbow because it's significant. And that tells us our hearings are going to be the best hearings, and it'll help the Committee do its work. There's no question we have and we will, the Chairman and I and the Committee, work together on veterans' issues.

I also want to thank Ernie Matsukawa from the Maui Vets Center. Also, Terri Garcia from the Office of Veterans Services in Maui, and Naomi Guardado from the J. Walter Cameron Center which we are in now, who have been working with my staff to coordinate these hearings. We greatly appreciate your hard work. So mahalo nui loa for what you have done.

[Applause.]

Senator AKAKA. My purpose in bringing the Committee to Hawaii for field hearings is to find out more about the state of VA care in Hawaii. I applaud the efforts of every VA employee in Hawaii. I also applaud our officials of the VA who have worked hard, in the region as well as nationally. Secretary Nicholson is relatively new, but has worked real hard in trying to do the best for our veterans across the country. There are many things that the VA does well in Hawaii. However, there is always room for improvement.

I want to hear about how we can help VA help Hawaii veterans. Today, and over this entire week, the Committee will examine the state of VA care in Hawaii. And I'm glad we're here on beautiful Maui with representatives from Molokai, and Lanai. As such, VA must tailor its strategy to reach all of Hawaii's veterans.

We know that the access for care for those living on what we call the neighbor islands—Kauai, Molokai, Lanai, Maui, and the Big Island—could be improved. As such, I developed a bill that would ensure a greater presence on the islands of Molokai and Lanai, which currently lack VA facilities altogether. And I'm sure we'll hear about that today.

A veteran living on either of these remote islands must either wait for a VA provider to visit, which is only 9 to 10 times a year for Molokai and 4 times a year for Lanai, or take it upon himself to get on Maui for clinical care, or to Oahu for treatment for a more serious condition.

Filling up the car with a tank of gas and driving across the State is obviously not even an option here. Inter-island air fare is more than $200, and besides that, we don't have bridges between the islands. So veterans have difficulty getting reimbursed for these expenses, which also include rental cars and hotels. Many veterans who cannot afford these costs must choose to forgo care as a result.

Even when a VA provider finally comes to one of these remote islands, they have no tele-medicine equipment—this from a Department that is renowned for their computerized medical records and technologies. I'm sure all of you know that healthcare provided by VA is No. 1 in the Nation by the Veterans Administration. That's a fact.

VA also needs to revamp its beneficiary travel program. This benefit is one that is highly valued by many veterans, especially those on fixed incomes. Unfortunately, there has not been an increase in the benefit for some time. In 2001, VA found that the current allowances under this program were not sufficient to begin to deal with high gas prices. Yet 4 years later, the increase was never put forward.

We are privileged to have all of our witnesses with us this morning. We will hear first from veterans' representatives from Maui, Lanai, and Molokai. It is vitally important that you share your thoughts with us so that we know how to help VA help you and the rest of Hawaii's veterans. VA officials will respond to the concerns laid out by the previous panel. That's a response not only on the national and regional level, but the local level as well, State level, and on our congressional level.

Finally, I want to address the fact that there are many veterans who are here today and who want to testify. We want to hear from you. And I'm glad to have met some of you before the meeting outside, because some of you would have liked to testify. But we can't hear everybody. Unfortunately, this is a problem, and we cannot accommodate everyone's request.

However, we are accepting written testimony for the record. So you can rest assured that we will read your written testimony. If you have brought written testimony with you, please give it to the Committee staff who are located in the back of the room—they're raising their hands back there.

But if you do not have a written statement, but would like to submit something, our staff is in the back of the room to assist you with that also. In addition, the Committee staff is joined by VA staff who can respond to the questions, concerns, and comments that you raise, and will also be at that table.

Once again, mahalo nui loa to all of you who are in attendance today, and I look forward to hearing from today's witnesses.

Senator AKAKA. We welcome the first panel here today. I'm sure you're all familiar to the folks here in the tri-island County, the three islands: The first one is Rogelio Evangelista, who's the—as I call you, just raise your hand—the President, Maui Veterans Council. Rogelio. I've got to tell you, Rogelio was not supposed to be here today. He was supposed to have an operation. But he postponed that to be here. Thank you very much.

Also, Larry Helm, the well-known President, Molokai Veterans Caring for Veterans.

Roy Kekahuna, Doctor, District Director, Blinded Veterans Association. We're glad to have you, Roy.

Dwight "Lui" Obado, organizer of the Lanai Veterans Organization, is here.

We're delighted to have you folks. We want to hear what you have to say. You're welcome to come sit at the table. We're delighted to have you folks here. You will testify in the order you were introduced. So mahalo nui loa to you, and you can begin.

STATEMENT OF ROGELIO EVANGELISTA, PRESIDENT, MAUI VETERANS COUNCIL

Mr. EVANGELISTA. Thank you, Senator. Before we go on, if we can have a prayer first. Mario? Are you here? Can you lead us in a prayer? And after that, maybe we can have a Pledge of Allegiance. Will you stand.

[Opening prayer and Pledge of Allegiance.]

Chairman CRAIG. Please proceed.

Mr. EVANGELISTA. Mr. Chairman, Larry Craig, Senator Akaka, and distinguished Members of the Senate Veterans' Affairs Committee, Veterans Administration Pacific Islands Healthcare System Director General Hastings and staff, thank you for giving me this opportunity to come before you today to discuss the state of the VA care in Hawaii, home to more than 110,000 veterans, and especially for the more than 10,000 veterans living in the county of Maui, which comprises the 3 islands of Maui, Molokai, and Lanai out of the 8 islands that make up the State of Hawaii, which are all separated by the ocean.

The excellent medical efforts of the Maui CBOC, the Community Based Outreach Clinic, with the support of the Spark Matsunaga Center on Oahu and the Tripler Army Medical Center, have been extraordinary. I would at this time like to take a moment to stress the unique nature of healthcare here on Maui, Molokai, and Lanai, and to also include Kauai and Hawaii.

The first, by being on the State Veterans Advisory Board for over 9 years and on the VAMROC, which is the Veterans Administration Medical and Regional Office Center, Advisory Board for over 5 years, and as a disabled veteran, I have understood the stress and witness the bureaucracy the veterans are faced when receiving healthcare from the Veterans Administration.

They must be able to pass the means test by having limited income jointly with their spouse so that if they need to go to Oahu or the mainland for specialized care that is not service-connected, they will be provided airline transportation. And this is for any veteran with less than 30 percent disability that uses the VA healthcare system as their primary healthcare.

If the veteran does not qualify on the means test and he or she has a disability of less than 30 percent, then the veteran must pay their own transportation to go to Oahu or the mainland. Veterans on the mainland can drive to the VA hospitals and not worry about passing any means test. VA states it's cheaper to have the exam or procedure done on Oahu with the veteran paying about $145 for a round-trip ticket instead of having the veteran see a local provider on the island that he or she resides on. Veterans' bills are even being sent to collection agencies because the VA takes so long on paying for services from outside providers.

Second, as I look at our aging veteran population, there are 100 percent disabled veterans in nursing homes on Maui with the families paying over $7,000 per month for their healthcare at those nursing homes, plus their medications. It's hard for the families to send them to Oahu to the Center for Aging, and there will be no family support because they can't fly to Oahu every day to see the veteran. Is it possible for VA to do a partnership with Hale Makua, a nursing home on the island of Maui, for the veterans living on Maui? Why is Hawaii and Alaska the last two States that do not have any VA hospital? What happened to a Federal mandate that states that there should be a VA hospital in each State?

Third, our CBOCs on all the neighbor islands, even with the experienced and dedicated staff, they are underpaid in comparisom with the mainland VA staff. And they are also overworked. We need more staffing and we need more office space on Maui and on the other neighbor islands. On Maui, if the VA can buy out the building that CBOC is located in and the vacant lot next to the building and look at expanding services with more staff we now have volunteers, but they are limited in the scope off work that they can perform. And we need more specialized equipment, especially for telemedicine.

There is now one full-time doctor 5 days a week, one part-time doctor 4 days a week. We need to upgrade our staff to provide the best possible care for our veterans. Right now it takes so long to get an appointment to see the doctor for routine or specialized care. The doctor has to come in from Oahu or the mainland.

In order to provide ongoing care to veterans, first, the Government must realize that veterans' healthcare is part of the cost of war, and that the Government needs to provide enough funding for VA healthcare to all veterans. Second, the Veterans Administration, along with the Government, must identify and develop programs and use today's technologies to help veterans in their daily lives, especially for our disabled veterans.

Combinations of advanced healthcare using new technologies will greatly help all of our veterans, and make their recoveries possible and the long-term relationship of being accepted back into society. I ask you, why is VA funding always the lowest priority in our Government, when we, the veterans, made our country the greatest Nation in the world?

Fourth, many of our veterans are suffering from some sort of physical or mental disability and would rather alienate themselves from anything to do with the Veterans Administration due to many contributing factors. All the red tape that they must go through to even start to file their claim, something that happened over 30 years ago, and it is just being addressed today because of the veteran's health status, be it physical or mental. And this is all due to different contributing factors of the veteran's healthcare.

Veterans are being informed to get collaborating [sic] evidence from other veterans that served with them and might know something regarding the veteran's condition or of an incident that occurred. Most of the veterans don't know where these other veterans are now living, and some of them just don't want to get involved. But there are records that the military have, so why can't the Veterans Administration get those records to collaborate [sic] the veteran's claim?

Fifth, veterans are now paying $7 co-payment on drugs and medication, and the VA is also at this time exploring the idea of raising the co-payment on drugs for veterans that are being prescribed for non-service-connected medical problems. These veterans are on very limited financial support due to their physical and mental conditions being attributed to their military career in one way or another.

They answered our Nation's call when they were needed. Why can't our Nation now help them in their time of need? I ask and plead with you, the Members of the Veterans' Affairs Committee, to lobby your constituents and help our Nation's veterans lead fruitful and dignified lives.

Sixth, the vocational rehab program that tried to help veterans in training them for a vocation that they can excel in is great. But now there are so much restraints being placed on being able to qualify, and the approval all now comes from Washington, DC and not done here locally like it used to be.

There is so much paperwork going back and forth, and it takes such a long time, sometimes longer than 6 months for approval if it does get approved, and by that time the veteran has already lost interest and have given up on the system.

When you apply for vocational rehabilitation, you will need specialized and long-term counseling and support from your case worker here and not from somebody from Washington that knows you only as a number, with no personal knowledge of all your special needs as you continue with your studying. And this will be due to the type of medications that you are being prescribed by the doctor, so the doctors and your case worker need to be informed on your physical and mental condition so that you can be successful in pursuing your vocational training.

There are veterans here on Maui that don't even know of certain benefits that they may be qualified to apply for due to their physical and mental disabilities. Vocational rehabilitation is a part of medical. It's due to your physical condition.

Seventh, our veterans now from the Gulf War and those returning from Iraq are now at this time being diagnosed with illness not yet known. We need to expand our technology to help these veterans and their families so they can cope with their personal problems.

By extending our medical staff at our clinics, it won't take 2 or 3 months or more for an x-ray, MRI, and other specialized tests that need to be done to identify the cause of the veteran's illness or his disabling injuries so the veteran can be placed in various programs in mental, physical, or vocational areas so the veteran can start to lead a fruitful and normal life in our society.

Eighth, single veterans are being discharged from the hospital, but still are not able to care for themselves, and they can't get any home care since cases are so backlogged, they have to go on a waiting period. We need a home care nurse here on the island of Maui and Molokai and Lanai.

And also after hours, if you need to go to emergency and use your VA card, about 2 or 3 months later you get a notice from the VA that your emergency visit was not covered since it was not related to a disability or since the attending physician stated that you were OK on the checkup at emergency.

On behalf of the veterans of the State of Hawaii, especially the county of Maui, and all their families, I would like to ask all the Members of the Senate Committee on Veterans' Affairs, along with the Veterans Administration Pacific Islands Healthcare System Director and staff, for their support of these men and women who committed a part of their lives and well-being to defend and protect our great Nation, the United States of America.

Will the Committee now, along with their constituents, give their full support to our veterans and provide a healthcare that is second to none and a budget to surpass the costs of administering the greatest healthcare to all our veterans.

Thank you. May God bless America, its people, the armed forces, and especially its veterans and their families.

[Applause.]

[The prepared statement of Mr. Evangelista follows:]

PREPARED STATEMENT OF ROGELIO EVANGELISTA, PRESIDENT, MAUI VETERANS COUNCIL

Mr. Chairman Larry Craig, Senator Akaka, and distinguished Members of the Senate Veterans Affairs Committee, VAPIHCS Director Gen. Hastings and Staff, thank you for giving me this opportunity to come before you today to discuss the state of VA care in Hawaii, home to more than 110,000 veterans and especially for the more than 10,000 veterans living in the County of Maui, which comprises the three islands of Maui, Molokai, and Lanai out of the eight islands that make up the State of Hawaii which are all separated by the ocean.

The excellent medical efforts of the Maui CBOC [Community Based Outreach Clinic] with the support of the Spark Matsunaga Center on Oahu, and the Tripler Army Medical Center have been extra ordinary. I would at this time like to take a moment to stress the unique nature of health care here on Maui, Molokai, Lanai, and to also include Kauai, and Hawaii.

First, by being on the State Veterans Advisory Board for over 9 years and on the VAMROC [Veterans Administration Medical & Regional Office Center] Advisory Board for over 5 years and as a Disabled Veteran, I have understood the stress and witnessed the bureaucracy that Veterans are faced when receiving health care from the Veterans Administration. They must be able to pass the Means Test by having limited income jointly with their spouse, so that if they need to go to Oahu, or the Mainland for specialized care that is not service connected, they will be provided airline transportation, and this are for any Veteran with less than 30 percent disability that uses the VA Health Care System as their Primary Health care. If the Veteran do not qualify on the Means Test and he or she has a disability of less than 30 percent then the Veteran must pay their own transportation to go to Oahu, or the mainland. Veterans on the Mainland can drive to the VA hospitals and not worry about passing any Means Test. VA states it is cheaper to have the exam or procedure done on Oahu with the Veteran paying about $145.00 for a round trip ticket, instead of having the Veteran see a local provider on the island that he resides on. Veteran bills are even being sent to collection agencies because the VA takes so long on paying for the services from outside providers.

Second, as I look at our aging Veteran population, there are 100 percent disabled veterans in Nursing homes on Maui with the families paying over $7,000.00 per month for their health care at those Nursing homes plus their medications and its hard for the families to send them to Oahu to the Center for Aging and there will be no family support because they can't fly to Oahu everyday to see the Veteran. Is it possible for the VA to do a partnership with Hale Makua, a Nursing home on the Island of Maui for the Veterans living on Maui. Why is Hawaii and Alaska the last 2 states that do not have any VA hospital, what happened to a Federal mandate that states that there should be a VA hospital in each state.

Third, our CBOC's, on all the neighbor islands, even with the experienced and dedicated staff, they are underpaid in comparing with the mainland VA staff, and they are also overworked, we need more staffing and we need more office space, on Maui, if the VA can buy out the building that CBOC is located in and the vacant lot next to the building and look at expanding services with more staff, we now have volunteers but they are limited in the scope of work that they can perform. There is now one full time doctor 5 days a week, one part time doctor 4 days a week, we need to upgrade our staff to provide the best possible care for our Veterans, right now it takes so long to get an appointment to see the doctor, for routine or specialized care, the doctor has to come in from Oahu or the mainland. In order to provide ongoing care to Veterans, first, the government must realize that Veterans health care are part of the cost of war and that the government needs to provide enough funding for VA health care to all Veterans, second, the Veterans Administration along with the government must identify and develop programs and use today technologies to help Veterans in their daily lives, especially for our disabled veterans. Combinations of advanced health care using new technologies will greatly help all of our veterans and make their recoveries possible and the long term relationship of being accepted back into society. Why is VA funding always the lowest priority in our government, when we the Veterans made our country the greatest Nation in the world.

Fourth, many of our Veterans are suffering from some sort of physical or mental disability and would rather alienate themselves from anything to do with the Veterans Administration due to many contributing factors. All the red tape that they must go through to even start to file their claim, something that happened over 30 years ago and it is just being addressed today because of the Veterans health status, be it physical or mental, Veterans are being informed to get collaborating evidence from other Veterans that served with them and might know something regarding the Veterans conditions or of an incident that occurred. Most of this Veterans don't know where these other veterans are now living and some of them just don't want to get involved, but there are records that the military have so why can't the Veterans Administration get those records to collaborate the Veterans claim.

Fifth, Veterans are now paying $7.00 co-payment on drugs and medication and the VA is also at this time exploring the idea of raising the co-payment on drugs for Veterans that are being prescribed for non-service connected medical problems, and these Veterans are living on very limited financial support due to their physical and mental conditions being attributed to their military career in one way or another. They answered our Nations call when they were needed, why can't our Nation now help them in their time of need, I ask and plead with you the members of the Veterans Affairs Committee to lobby your constituents and help our Nation's Veterans lead fruitful and dignified lives.

Sixth, the Vocational rehabilitation program that try to help Veterans in training them for a Vocation that they can excel in is great, but now there are so much restraints being placed on being able to qualify and the approval all now comes from Washington D.C. and not done here locally like it used to be. There is so much paper work going back and forth and it takes such a long time sometimes longer than 6 months for approval if it does get approved and by that time the Veteran has already lost interest and have given up on the system. When you apply for Vocational rehabilitation you will need specialized and long term counseling and support from your case worker here and not from somebody from Washington that knows you only as a number with no personal knowledge of all your special needs as you continue with your studies. There are Veterans here on Maui that don't even know of certain benefits that they may be qualified to apply for due to their physical and mental disabilities.

On behalf of the Veterans of the State of Hawaii, especially the County of Maui and all their Families, I would like to ask all the Members of the Senate Committee on Veterans Affairs, along with the VAPIHCS Director and Staff for their support of these men and women who committed a part of their lives and well being to defend and protect our great Nation, the United States of America. Will the committee now along with their constituents give their full support to our Veterans and provide a health care that is second to none and a budget to surpass the costs of administering the greatest health care to our heroes.

Thank you, may God Bless America, its people, the Armed Forces, and especially its Veterans and their Families.

Senator AKAKA. Thank you very much, Rogelio.

Larry.

STATEMENT OF LARRY HELM, PRESIDENT, MOLOKAI VETERANS CARING FOR VETERANS

Mr. HELM. Good morning, fellow veterans. I'd also say a special mahalo to our group from Molokai that got up at 4 this morning to catch the ferry to come over here for this.

[Applause.]

Mr. HELM. Senator Larry Craig, Chairman, Honorable Senator Danny Akaka, aloha kakahiaka to you and your staff. Welcome to Hawaii nei and to the island Maui. My name is Larry Helm, a heavy combat Vietnam veteran. I represent 345 Molokai veterans from all wars and conflicts. From the vsn of a Patsy Bird, the Molokai Veterans Caring for Veterans Center, Koa Kahiko, which means "strong, wise, ancient warrior," formed 4 years ago mainly for veterans to have a voice and address concerns on the island of Molokai.

Because we are an island in the Maui County surrounded by water, we therefore have been many challenges to get services for Molokai veterans. Today, the Veterans Administration is doing a lot more for the Molokai veterans. I thank you and ask you to please continue. I'm sure that there are a lot of rural "Molokais" throughout this country that face the challenges of caring for veterans.

Molokai has many combat Vietnam veterans that are finally getting help. The island has a population of 7,000 residents, and has contributed to this country greatly. We have a memorial stone in the middle of town naming 10 World War II, 6 Korean, and 5 Vietnam veterans who lost their lives for this country. There is a wall in Washington, DC with over 58,000 names of my brothers and sisters killed in action in country in Vietnam, but we do not have a wall for over 100,000 that prematurely died from wounds related to combat—Agent Orange, chronic PTSD, physical wounds, et cetera. This issue has been sanitized.

In the last year on Molokai, Koa Kahiko lost 5 Vietnam veterans. Spencer Eldridge, 56 years old, died 3 weeks ago. He handled Agent Orange on a ship outside the Tonkin Gulf. Three of our deceased veterans had just started to receive their service-connected disability benefits. The Molokai community has over 40 men and women who have served and are serving today in Afghanistan and Iraq.

I speak for past veterans, but essentially for those veterans who will return from the Middle East to Molokai. I emphasize the importance of continuing and improving the mental and physical healthcare they deserve. All service-connected claims must be efficiently and hastily processed sooner, not later.

The Molokai veteran community says thank you. The VA has certified Dr. Hafermann, a resident of Molokai, to practice on Molokai alongside with the medical team from Maui. I'd just like Dr. Hafermann to stand up. He's a colonel who used to be in charge of Travis Air Force Base.

[Applause.]

Mr. HELM. I ask to have more psychological help for our veterans on Molokai. It takes 6 months to get an appointment with Dr. McNamara, who is the Mother Teresa for the veterans, and her time is limited.

[Applause.]

Mr. HELM. We need more of her or hire two more Dr. McNamaras. Dr. Springer, a psychiatrist, will start this month. Mahalo.

To have an inpatient nurse help for older Molokai veterans.

We need a mini-honor guard burial service for service-connected veterans. Every veteran deserves that honor.

To not repeat the process that led us to lose many of our Vietnam veterans' lives, who did not get psychological help because of PTSD—suicide, despondence, hopelessness, deterioration of their body. In combat, one size does not fit all. Why would you want to revisit the studying of PTSD when the psychiatric community has studied this scientifically from all wars and has agreed that is a serious, permanent disorder that affects many veterans. I hope the Government does not water down the treatment for this mental disorder because of budget restraints, especially for our returning veterans.

To please continue providing veterans' organizations the opportunity to testify for the veterans' affairs. We heard Senator [sic] Buyer wanted to stop the VFW, DMV, the American Legion, et cetera, from giving testimony. That is absolutely not acceptable.

Starting a national—I suggest starting a national low interest credit union and credit card service for service-connected veterans and all other veterans, it could be a profitable and honorable thing to do for the veterans.

That spouses of 100 percent service-connected veterans qualify to receive their husband or wife's benefits 5 years rather than 10 years. Many veterans die prematurely and leave their spouse empty.

Senator Craig, Senator Akaka, mahalo for your time and the opportunity to testify here this morning, and hope you consider all that I have said. In my opinion, veterans are the soul of this country. The American people required that it be mandatory that the Congress provide whatever budget is needed to care for the veterans.

May Akua bless you and the United States of America. Aloha, aloha no.

[Applause.]

[The prepared statement of Mr. Helm follows:]

PREPARED STATEMENT OF LARRY HELM, PRESIDENT, MOLOKAI VETERANS
CARING FOR VETERANS

Aloha Kakahiaka (Good Morning) to you and your staff. Welcome to Hawaii nei and to the island of Maui. My name is Larry Helm, a heavy combat Vietnam Veteran. I represent 345 Molokai Veterans from all wars and conflict. From the vision of Patsy Bird, the Molokai Veterans Caring for Veterans Center-Koa Kahiko (strong, wise, ancient warrior) formed 4 years ago mainly for Veterans to have a voice and address concerns on the island of Molokai.

Because we are an island in Maui County surrounded by water, there have been many challenges to get services for Molokai Veterans. Today the Veterans Administration is doing a lot more for the Molokai Veterans. I thank you and ask you to please continue. I'm sure that there are a lot of rural "Molokais" throughout this country that face the challenges of caring for the veterans. Molokai has many combat Vietnam veterans that are finally getting help. The island has a population of 7,000 residents and has contributed to our country greatly. We have a memorial stone in the middle of town naming ten World War II, six Korean, and five Vietnam Veterans who lost their lives for this country.

There is a wall in Washington DC with over 58,000 names of my brothers and sisters killed in action in country in Vietnam but we do no have a wall for over 100,000 that prematurely died from wounds related to combat i.e. agent orange, chronic PTSD, physical wounds, etc. This issue has been sanitized. In the last year on Molokai, Koa Kahiko lost five Vietnam veterans. Eldridge Spencer, 56 years old, died 3 weeks ago from leukemia due to agent orange exposure. Three of the deceased veterans had just started to receive their service connected disability benefits. The Molokai Community has over 40 men/women who have served and are serving today in Afghanistan and Iraq.

I speak for past Veterans but especially for those veterans who will return from the Middle East to Molokai. I emphasize the importance of continuing and improving the mental and physical health-care they deserve. All service connected claims must be efficiently and hastily processed sooner not later.

The Molokai Veteran Community says "thank you". The VA has certified Dr. Havelman, a resident of Molokai, to practice on Molokai along side the medical team from Maui.

I ask:

• to have more psychological help for veterans on Molokai. It takes 6 months to get an appointment. Dr. McNamara is the Mother Theresa for the veterans and her time is limited. We need more of her or hire two more Dr. McNamaras. Dr. Springer, the psychiatrist will start this month. Mahalo.

• to have inpatient nurse help for older Molokai veterans.

• for a mini honor guard burial service for service connected veterans. Every veteran deserves the honor.

• to not repeat the process that led to the loss of many Vietnam veteran lives who did not get psychological help because of PTSD (suicide, despondence, hopelessness, and deterioration of their body). In combat, one size does not fit all. Why would you want to revisit the studying of PTSD when the psychiatric community has studied this scientifically from all wars and has agreed that PTSD is a serious permanent disorder that affects many veterans. I hope the government does not water down the treatment for this mental disorder because of budget restraints; especially for the returning Veterans.

• To please continue providing Veteran organizations the opportunity to testify for veterans affairs. We heard Senator Buyer wanted to stop VFW, DMV, etc. from giving testimony. That is absolutely not acceptable.

I suggest:

• starting a national veteran low interest credit union and credit card service for connected veterans and other veterans. It could be a profitable and honorable thing to do for our veterans.

• that spouses of 100 percent service connected veterans qualify to receive their husband/wife veteran benefits 5 years rather than 10 years. Many veterans die prematurely and leave their spouse empty.

Mahalo for your time and the opportunity to testify here this morning and hope you consider all that I have said. In my opinion, Veterans are the soul of this country. The American people require that it be mandatory that Congress provide whatever budget is needed to care for Veterans. May Akua bless you and the United States of America.

Aloha, aloha no.

Senator AKAKA. Mahalo. Mahalo, Larry.

And now we'll hear from Dr. Kekahuna.

STATEMENT OF ROY W. KEKAHUNA, PHD, DISTRICT DIRECTOR, BLINDED VETERANS ASSOCIATION

Dr. KEKAHUNA. Mr. Chairman and distinguished Members of the Committee, thank you for the opportunity to come before you to discuss the care of blinded veterans in general, and in specific, the needs of the blinded veterans in the State of Hawaii.

By way of introduction, I represent 10 Western States. In August, I will represent Hawaii and Alaska. Idaho, Mr. Chairman, happens to be one of the States in my District. I have 18 regional groups. Hawaii's regional group is currently defunct, so that's one of the reasons they asked me to come back to Hawaii and put it together.

Showing my background, I was born and raised here in the islands, originally from Molokai. My ancestor was the King of Maui; is interred on the island of Maui. His name was Alapai Nui in the ancient history of the Hawaiian islands. So there is a lot here for me in the State. That's why I'm here today. I have been to three blind centers, so I know what the blinded veterans of the State of Hawaii really need and deserve. I currently live in Las Vegas, and

I have been to the Blind Center, so I know what the blinded veterans of the State really need.

I would like to take a moment to stress that blindness is a catastrophic event in a veteran's life. Immediately, the veteran loses his or her independence. The uniqueness of this situation is that for the rest of this veteran's life, they will need assistance during 25 to 80 percent of their daily activities.

Another unique feature with a good percentage of the blinded veterans is that they have dual sensory loss (for example, hearing and visual loss). I have both hearing and eye problems from my injuries in Vietnam. Besides having vision and hearing problems, many of the blinded veterans have dual disabilities, such as the loss of use of an arm. I'm sure Senator Inouye could talk to that, as well as anybody else.

To give everybody an idea of what we have to go through in our life, if you'll all close your eyes. Keep them closed. Reach with your right hand for the left hand of the person next to you. Pretty hard to do, isn't it? Well, welcome to my world.

I use the Veterans Administration healthcare facilities for my medical services. Most area's of my medical experiences with VA have been favorable. Veterans Administration's care for their blinded veterans is behind the curve.

Veterans Administration in general is behind the curve in care for their blinded veterans. Their care for the blinded veterans of the State of Hawaii is in the dark ages. I cite myself as an example. I came home from Vietnam totally blind. There were no low vision services in the local Veterans Administration. Today, there is still no low vision services in VA, almost 40 years later. Blinded veterans of the State of Hawaii are less than stepchildren. I believe that this is criminal treatment of Hawaii blinded veterans.

Currently, the VA in Hawaii provides a part-time Vision Impairment Services Team Coordinator, called a VIST. The coordinator is responsible for case management of all blind and legally blinded veterans. They do not train blinded veterans. The VIST coordinator works only 5 percent of her work period on blinded veterans. This is inefficient for the workload.

I'll give you an example because I did some research before I got here. There currently 50 veterans in the vision program. In the VA, there are 200 blinded veterans registered with eye clinic in the State of Hawaii. In the area of high risk, there are 700 veterans currently enrolled in the VA Eye Clinic. These numbers only reflect the veterans who have come out of the woodwork, and realize that they are due these benefits.

Ho'opono, the State of Hawaii's vocational rehabilitation, is the only low vision/blind service currently available to veterans. It is VA's responsibility to care for the veterans as it promised. The blinded veterans of the State of Hawaii need your support to gain equal treatment, which their brother and sister veterans of the other 49 States have.

As an example—some more research—VA outlying clinics are not equipped to assist visual impairment. State Rehab for the Blind is a 9-month program, where the VA has better programs located on the continent. There are no housing facilities to go with this. Our island veterans, such as people on Maui, Molokai, and Lanai have an expense that is insurmountable just to get there. The non-service-connected veterans have no chance unless they pay for it out of their pocket presently.

I applaud the VA and the Department of Defense, DoD, partnership that they have here in Hawaii. Together they have the makings of a perfect harmony to service the blinded veterans. In this opportunity scenario, the Army Medical Detachment, AMMED, at Tripler Army Medical Center, TAMC, as it's called, can provide a full-time low vision doctor, while would provide a full-time VIST/Blind Rehabilitation Outreach Specialist, BROS.

The State of Hawaii's geographical island makeup supports the need of a VIST/BROS full-time specialist. The individual who operates from this position can provide both casework and training for the blinded veteran while on the different islands. I would highly recommend the creation of this position as soon as possible.

In the best of times and the best of situations, the blinded veteran should attend a VA Blind Rehabilitation Center. I notice that we have people here from Palo Alto, California who work at the Blind Rehab Center, and I applaud you. I am a graduate.

Ho'opono's program is 9 months long. Anybody on the outer islands, on all of the islands, who just have the transportation costs, make it almost inaccessible for them to attend. Blinded veterans on the island of Oahu currently have a place they can go for training. The VA should send other blinded veterans to the Blind Rehab Centers, or they should have specialists on each and every island to take care of these veterans.

I have experienced the excellent medical services provided at TAMC. I have been to four sessions at different Blind Rehabilitation Centers and received excellent training. I believe that it is important to fund the VA, Department of Defense medical facilities, and staff them properly. I don't care how good your facility is; if you are not staffed properly it will not work.

On behalf of blinded veterans and their families, the people of Hawaii, I thank the Members of this great institution for providing us with the funding and resources to take care of the finest men and women that I've had the pleasure to represent today. Thank you.

[Applause.]

[The prepared statement of Mr. Kekahuna follows:]

PREPARED STATEMENT OF ROY W. KEKAHUNA, PhD, DISTRICT DIRECTOR, BLINDED VETERANS ASSOCIATION

Mister Chairman and distinguished members of the committee, thank you for the opportunity to come before you today to discuss the care of blinded veterans in general, and in specific the needs of the blinded veterans in the State of Hawaii.

I would like to take a moment to stress that blindness is a catastrophic event in a veterans' life. Immediately the veteran loses his or her independence. The uniqueness of this situation is that for the rest of those veterans' lives, they will need assistance during 25 to 85 percent of their daily activities.

Another unique feature with a good percentage of the blinded veterans, is that they have dual sensory loss (for example, hearing and vision). Many of the blinded veterans have multiple disabilities (an example, loss of limbs).

A BRIEF DEMONSTRATION OF WHAT A BLIND VETERAN HAS TO GO THROUGH
TO DO A SIMPLE TASK

I use the Veterans Administration (VA) Health Care Facilities for my medical services. Most areas of my medical experiences with VA have been favorable; Veterans Administration's care for their blinded veterans is behind the curve.

Veterans Administration in general is behind the curve in care for their blinded veterans; their care for the blinded veterans of the State of Hawaii is in the dark ages. I cite myself as an example. I came home from Vietnam totally blind. There were no low vision services at the local Veterans Administration. Today, there is still no low vision specialist at the VA. Almost 40 years later, the blinded veterans of the State of Hawaii are less than a stepchild. I believe that this is criminal treatment of our Hawaii Blinded Veterans.

Currently the VA in Hawaii provides a part-time Vision Impairment Services Team Coordinator (VIST). The coordinator is responsible for the case management for all blind and legally blinded veterans. They do not train blinded veterans. The VIST coordinator in Hawaii works only 5 percent of her work period on blinded veterans cases. This is inefficient for the caseload.

Ho'opono, the state of Hawaii's vocational rehabilitation is the only low vision/blind service currently available to veterans. It is VA's responsibility to care for its veterans as promised. The blinded veterans of the State Hawaii need your support to gain equal treatment, which their brother and sister blinded veterans of the other 49 States receive.

I applaud the VA and the Department of Defense (DOD) partnership that they have here in Hawaii. Together they have the makings for a perfect harmony to service the blinded veterans. In this opportune scenario the Army Medical Department (AMMED) at Tripler Army Medical Center (TAMC) can provide a full time low vision doctor while VA would provide a full time VIST/Blind Rehabilitation Outreach Specialist (BROS).

The State of Hawaii's geographical island makeup supports the need of a VIST-BROS full time specialist. The individual who operates from this position can provide both casework and training for the blinded veteran while on the different islands. I would highly recommend the creation of this position as soon as possible.

In the best of times and in the best situation the blinded veteran should attend a VA Blind Rehabilitation Centers (BRC). The closest BRC for Hawaii's' blinded veterans is Palo Alto, CA. The current configuration of the blind services training at Ho'opono only works for those veterans residing on the island of Oahu. There are no resident facilities for the other island veterans.

I have experienced the excellent medical services provided at TAMC. I have been to four sessions at different BRC's and received excellent training. I believe that it is important to fund the VA, DOD Medical facilities, and staff them properly to support our current blinded veteran population and the next generation of blinded veteran that is already here from the conflicts/wars that we fight. This means keeping the promise.

On behalf of the blinded veterans and their families, I thank the members of this great institution for providing us with the funding and resources to take care of the finest men and women that I have had the honor to represent here today.

Senator AKAKA. Before I call on Lui, I just want to say something about what Larry mentioned while he was testifying, and that was he said aloha kakahiaka. And for those of you who don't know Hawaiian, what he said was good morning. Kakahiaka is "morning." Thank you, Larry.

And now we'll hear from Lui, Lui Obado.

STATEMENT OF DWIGHT "LUI" OBADO, ORGANIZER, LANAI VETERANS ORGANIZATION

Mr. OBADO. Hello. Thank you, everybody. Thank you for attending. I appreciate your calling—bringing Lanai over here. Welcome all to Lanai.

I know the weather in Washington. I was stationed in Aberdeen Proving Ground, and I also was stationed in Fort Lee, Virginia. I know your weather, and I love being away from it.

[Laughter.]

Mr. OBADO. So welcome to Lanai. This is a good day to be coming to Hawaii. This is a good day to be in Hawaii.

Now, let me tell you how it is where the rubber meets the road. We are the ones—Molokai and Lanai are the ones—that are really hurting. OK? Let me tell you about how we're really hurting.

First off, we have post-traumatic syndrome cases in Lanai. They affect our wives. Our wives is affected by getting wife abuse. And they don't want to come to Lanai because they don't have their money reimbursed.

We make an arrangement. We pay our own arrangement for our boat from Lanai to Lahaina. Then from Lahaina, we should catch that DAV van. All right? But if we get the DAV van, the DAV van supposedly picks us up at Lahaina and bring us to Kahului. But the DAV van shows up only 40 percent of the time, and we have to wait a whole hour at Lahaina Airport—I mean, Lahaina Harbor—for us to make an arrangement and get a taxi if they don't show up. The taxi costs us, again, the average of $47 from Lahaina to Kahului.

Now, the DAV van driver hang up the keys at 1. If our appointment going to keep us after 1, then we've got to go through the people again and find a taxi and cost another $47 from Kahului back to Lahaina, and another $30 from Lahaina to Lanai. That's money out of our pockets that we can't claim. Right there. And that's [inaudible] to me, but [inaudible] and VA. And he gets there all the time. All the time. But it's money out of our pockets that we cannot claim.

And we're VA. We signed the dotted line to join the military. When we sign that dotted line, we put our lives on the line and we put our families on hold. And when we did that, we gave that 100—more than 110 percent. Now we've got to have the 110 percent back. We need that.

In Lanai, it's out of sight, out of mind. I wrote a Committee to say, reimburse us for our trip here to make this appointment. They said, no. You get a—make a fund-raising to support your trip to Maui, and [inaudible] or not. You know, I don't understand. You explain that to me. OK? If I am [inaudible], then this is the [inaudible] function, then you should be reimbursing us for our vote. But money out of our pockets.

I pay the dues for this organization. Money out of my own personal pocket for our organization. I don't have money back. None. OK? It's a lot of stuff that Lanai people pay out our pocket, and we don't have—we can't claim it back. Period.

Another one we can't claim it back is another health insurance, which is TRICARE. The VA clinic over here tells me—I'm going to give you my experience—tells me that they won't service me because I have health insurance. So I use my health insurance, which is TRICARE, because I'm a retired military. I use the TRICARE, and I get the bill. So I sent the bill to VA. VA said, no. You pay your bill.

All I wanted was a B–12 shot. That's all I wanted. All I want is them to bring a syringe to Lanai and use the medication that I brought from the mainland and give me a shot. And their answer, the VA answer, is no. Use your insurance. And I did, and did I claim it? I mean, did I get the money back? No. This is where the rubber meets the road.

Lanai, we all have the problem. The problem is sitting right there, too. You see all of us have come. We're all 100 percent disabled. We're all a Category 1. And for the VA clinic to tell us, Category 1 personnel, who is more than 100 percent disabled, tell me that they're not going to service me and for me to use my insurance? No. My insurance is for my wife and my son. I use the VA clinic system.

And now I come over here and they says, no. We won't service you. I'm a Category 1 personnel. What are you doing, you know? Don't you know your own regulations? So I am called—this VA hospital called me a troublemaker. I am not a troublemaker. I'm just asking you to read the regulation, understand your regulation, and do what you're supposed to be doing. That's what I am doing. So I'm a troublemaker. Oh well, you know?

I'm trying to stay on schedule here. I don't want to go over. So that's fine. I didn't bring any write-up.

Anyway, back—oh, I am dyslexic, ADD, and brain-injured. So— and I also wear a hearing aid. I don't have it on today because I didn't bring my spare with me. So I'm very dysfunctional. You see? I got a dysfunctional veteran hat: "Leave me alone."

[Laughter.]

Mr. OBADO. [Inaudible.] My permanent VA clinic is in Vancouver, Washington. When I come to Hawaii, I'm a visitor to Hawaii. But I'm helping all the veterans in Lanai because they are not getting the care I'm getting from the mainland. OK?

My care, I get it all from the mainland. And I come over here and I see Lanai don't have any kind of care. We have care once a month. OK? We have [inaudible] officer, which is Bill, come over here once a month. Once a month is not going to cut it for Lanai because Lanai, we need the veterans—like Bill, we need a veteran to sit down with Bill and do our claim. [Inaudible.] Once a month.

You know, if you live in Maui, just run down to the clinic. Make an appointment and run down to the clinic. What's it going to cost you? It costs you gas money. That's all. It costs us a boat trip, which is $60, a taxi fare, which is $47 one way, and they hang up the keys at 1, and then it costs us another $47 back this way. OK?

I'm 3 minutes over. Anyway, I want to let you guys know that I am the only one in all of Hawaii that [inaudible] the United States Army [inaudible]. And that's why I am so eager to help the veterans in Lanai to get something what is they deserve when they sign that dotted line. Thank you.

[Applause.]

[The prepared statement of Mr. Obado follows:]

PREPARED STATEMENT OF DWIGHT "LUI" OBADO, ORGANIZER, LANAI VETERANS ORGANIZATION

We respectfully call to your attention to the seriousness of the problem of Veterans medical care in Lanai Hawaii. We wish to emphasize the importance of the Veteran's Medical care of one of the most needed health benefit and vital to those veterans residing in Lanai.

Federal policymakers are unaware of the many challenges faced by Lanai veterans due to geography of our State. We would need to introduce a Bill to provide a new satellite clinics in both health-care and mental health service.

The agency also would have to improve mental health and substance abuse services in Lanai. We have a few veterans who are not right in their heads because of their war experiences. You would call this chronic sickness (PTSD). They have spaced out thoughts and attitudes. Even to a point of blacking out and getting an attack. Loosing tempers and yelling at their families and friends. One of our Veteran wife had to lock her self in the bedroom because her husband was yelling at her and stabbing the door with a knife. He is a Korean veterans and a Purple Heart recipient. I always have to go to his house when his wife calls me when he has his attacks and he always tells me he doesn't know what he was doing. He doesn't want to go to Maui for treatment because it costs him too much money and he had problems in the past of collecting his travel expense back from VA. See VA letter pertaining to his case and my travel case. The "red tape and bureaucracy" involve in obtaining any kind of medical care here in Lanai can be tough and frustrating to cope with.

I can readily appreciate the strain on the Federal budget; nevertheless, we ask that you consider giving us your consideration of a satellite clinics with both health-care and mental health service.

On behalf of the veterans' in Lanai Hawaii, We would like to thank you for helping us work together to accomplish our goal and what we cannot do alone. God Bless the United States of America for the U.S. Senate, Committee on Veterans' Affairs to helping us. Please show your patriotism and that you care for our veteran's. Please make the deference and love the country we veterans' kept free and great.

Chairman CRAIG. Lui, thank you very much for your testimony. I have a couple of questions, but I want to make a couple of observations prior to those questions.

First and foremost to all of you, we believe your testimony to be heartfelt and directed appropriately. Part of the reason we're here is to not only understand where there are problems, but also to create, where we can, a greater evenness of coverage and healthcare access.

And we also know that there are challenges. We can't have a veterans hospital everywhere. In fact, today, quite the opposite is happening across the country. Today, with technology, we're not building bricks and concrete any more as much as we used to. And no one else in the healthcare field is because of the use of technology.

I think, Larry, you mentioned, possibly you, Larry, telemedicine as an approach. That is only one of many that are allowing healthcare professionals to outreach in ways that heretofore have not—we've not been able to do in rural environments of the kind that you live in here or that my veterans live in Idaho.

There is no question we are being able to extend healthcare in areas where we could not before, or facilitate those who, as you said, have to travel by boat. In situations in my State, we have people who get in cars and drive 250 and 300 miles to gain access to VA healthcare.

So there are similar kinds of problems, and I think it's important that we hear those and that we attempt to resolve, where we can, those kinds of difficulties that do exist.

Let me say this because I am extremely proud of the work that has been done over time. There are a variety of illusions, and I use that word, illusion, as to what taxpayers and Congress are or are not doing for America's veterans.

But here's a reality: Of all the budgets that I look at, the one budget that has consistently had higher rates of increase over the last decade, over any other budget, has been the veterans' budget. Why? Because of the direct and open and obvious commitment that not only the Congress has, but we think Congress is reflective of America's concern.

You watched, I think, with great interest the debate we went through this past year. And we nearly doubled the budget as it was once proposed. It isn't a partisan issue. President Bush proposed a budget. President Clinton proposed different budgets. Congress disagreed, and put more money into it. And that is consistently the case.

Over the last decade, we've seen a near-average increase of 9 percent, on the whole, on an annualized basis, in the veterans' healthcare. If you'll notice today's press, healthcare costs this year inflated at a lower rate of about 9 percent.

We are not able to meet all of the needs or all of the perceived needs. We do have to establish priority. We do have to look at those who are in greater need and have less means within the veterans population to do so.

It is difficult for most who look at our Government who think, well, if you can spend money over there, why can't you spend money over here in a different area? Veterans' budgets, the VA budget, versus Health and Human Services, versus Agriculture, versus Defense, are very clear and separate budgets, and they are viewed as that. And they don't commingle.

And as much as we are—and I believe that to be—Danny and I, advocates for veterans, we have advocates there in Congress for all other areas of expenditures. And they fight as aggressively for their money as we do for your money.

And as a result, we're about to go through another budget cycle. The President will propose a budget. The Congress will look at it. This authorizing Committee that Danny and I serve on will look at the VA budget very, very closely. We will make recommendations to the Budget Committee. The Budget Committee will be looking at it. The Budget Committee will then lay out a level of expenditure based on what they think is necessary, and we will work the process down.

But there is a bottom line, and I'm very proud of that bottom line. That is that VA has been extremely well funded for the last decade as it compares to other areas of our Government. The only other area that we see larger increases is defense, and it's obvious to most of us why that's occurred, since 9/11, at least, in the last good number of years.

So as we work these issues through, and we will continue to do so. Not only do we work to get the money, but we also work to reestablish priorities or to look at where there are greater needs, to see if older services once offered are still legitimate, or if we opt to shift money to other areas and categories within VA healthcare, to do so.

Having said all that, Danny mentioned in his opening comments something that, again, both he and I are extremely proud of. Over the last several years, in numerous write-ups in national journals across the country, as a result of an analysis of quality care delivery, VA has come out No. 1.

I think if we think back just a few years, that was not the case. VA, when you as a veteran might have had alternative healthcare access, might have chosen that over VA. Today, that is simply not the case. As a result of us investing in VA healthcare and upping its overall quality, we've also accelerated the demand. Veterans have looked at it, when available, as an option or a selection of first choice in their healthcare.

Those are some of my observations as we work through this, that we are very proud of the VA healthcare system. We do recognize it as a quality healthcare delivery system. But gaining access, gaining service, rural environments, difficult geography, all of that complicates. There's no question about it.

And I must say that where it cannot be delivered in one location, is delivered in another, in a greater populated area, trying to therefore facilitate cost of transportation and movement so that veterans can get to those facilities. I don't think you can expect in remote environments comprehensive levels of care that oftentimes we experience in the more urban environments. It is simply a reality, although it's changing because of the technologies that are being allowed to us today.

Let me ask you, Dr. Roy, with your blind—your experience as an injured veteran and a blind veteran, you mentioned in your testimony that you've been to a number of VA blind rehabilitation facilities for training, or BRCs, as they are generally residential programs which require long stays away from family.

Dr. KEKAHUNA. Right.

Chairman CRAIG. And I'm sure you would agree that many veterans do not want to spend long days away from their families. That's a difficulty.

So the question would be: Do you believe that blind rehabilitation outpatient specialists are an adequate substitute to a residential program ? Or is the residential program of more benefit?

Dr. KEKAHUNA. I believe that the outreach program here in Hawaii would be most beneficial. In most instances, those veterans that can go to the Blind Rehabilitation Center should go there because it gives you the opportunity to become who you can be, all you can be, all in one place.

But because of the situation and the geographical location, blind outreach specialists would be most beneficial here immediately. Getting the veterans then onto the program to go forward to the BRC would be the next step because even after they get the basic training—at least they can survive at home—with the outreach program, then the VA should get them to the blind center so that they can get all of the equipment and the education that's needed to facilitate their lives.

I went to Hines in 1968. I went to Palo Alto because, through the grace of God and medical science, I've had vision back in one eye, and in 1988 I became legally blind again. And becoming legally blind, I was able to go to—to Palo Alto because they had good computer access to get my PhD. So that's why I went to Palo Alto, because at that time, even that was a scary place. Let me tell you why.

[Inaudible]. So by the time I went back to college and 6 months later, my computer was out of date. It's no longer that way, and that's a blessing for the veterans that go there now because they get the latest equipment and help them do what they need to do for their lives.

But outreach, yes, by far in this State.

Chairman CRAIG. Well, I thank you for that. I will disagree with that observation. I think that clearly to gain those course skills that you need, you need that clinical/student/classroom environment that, by the nature of its costs and realities, can only be put in certain locations. And we simply have to take the veteran to that location instead of expect that kind of facility in others.

Danny, let me turn to you. And again, gentlemen, your statements have become a part of the official record of the Committee. We thank you for your time and your commitment. Your work as advocates of veterans, that's greatly appreciated. You've been loudly heard today. Thank you.

[Applause.]

Senator AKAKA. Thank you very much, Mr. Chairman, for your remarks about the system. And I want to tell you that, as I mentioned, that working with Larry has been great. We together have been looking at better ways to try to service the veterans.

And with your kind of help, with your testimony in Hawaii and elsewhere, this will help us do that, as I mentioned in my remarks. You can help us to help you. This is what we're trying to do here. So Larry and I will continue to work hard on this Committee and try to take care of some of the problems that we hear, not only in Hawaii but across the country.

I'd like to ask a question of Mr. Helm, of Larry. In your testimony, you state that Molokai's veterans must wait 6 months to receive psychiatric care. Can you tell me about some of the problems that arise when veterans have to wait so long for care?

Mr. HELM. Senator, we do have a large population of Vietnam veterans, and because for many years the VA is finally catching up getting these veterans on line to get mental health, there's quite a few of them.

And Dr. McNamara just has so much time. She comes up there twice a month now. She used to come up once a month. So to see 5, 6, 7, 10 patients a day in an 8-hour or how many hours she's out on the island—she's got to come back in the afternoon; she comes in the morning—there's not enough. So sometimes it causes problems. The veterans get impatient. There's, you know, some problems at home and stuff like that. But it's been an ongoing thing for many years.

So if we could get Dr. McNamara a little bit more, it probably could fill the void. It's, I think, 5 months? If a guy goes to you, 3 months to 5 months? Yeah. It's down to 3 months now that she's coming twice a month. So if we could get her three times a month, that might mean more guys could get the help that they need.

Senator AKAKA. Mahalo for your response.

Mr. Obado, Lui, I was especially concerned to hear that veterans may not travel from Lanai to Maui for treatment because of what you said and issues they have collecting back money from travel reimbursement. And you have covered this pretty well.

My only question to you would be: Do you have an idea on how that could be done better?

Mr. OBADO. I think that ideally it would be better to have a satellite clinic in Lanai so they can, even through television, talk to another veteran doctor, and use our Straub Clinic, our doctor in the

Straub Clinic, to have a satellite clinic, and they can talk to a VA clinic through a satellite.

We have a doctor, Dr. Gasper. He used to be a doctor to a VA clinic. So he knows what it takes to help a veteran. And we have one on there. But he can't do it, because now he's a doctor for the Straub Clinic. But if he had the camera to talk to another veteran doctor, then we can go to the clinic ourselves. Instead of coming all the way to Maui, we can go straight to the Straub Clinic and the doctor there can just go to the television and discuss with another veteran doctor, and then that veteran will be helped.

Senator AKAKA. Thank you. Mahalo for your mana'o.

[Applause.]

Senator AKAKA. Larry, to buildupon Lui's statement, can you please explain the obstacles that a veteran must overcome to travel from Molokai to Maui for care? I understand that the ferry runs during the morning and evening rush hours and arrives on the western side of Maui near Lahaina town. So can you——

Mr. HELM. Yes, Senator. We do have a ferry that comes every day. We do have Island Air that flies from an airport. And the cost of Island Air is $216 round trip for us to come over here for care.

But very difficult sometimes to get the VA to tie in with the veterans' timeframe to get a flight and coordinate the appointment here. That's been the difficulty [inaudible].

Paperwork. Sometimes the paperwork did not get in, or the VA thought that they are going to Honolulu when he's supposed to come to Maui. And there's a lot of mix-ups like that. That could be solved if there was a little bit more efficiency there for the Molokai vets.

Also, now that we are having a doctor from on island there, and now that we're having or supposedly getting a psychiatrist, we also need an outreach counselor. We lost Robert Lewis, so we need an outreach counselor to come to Molokai on a regular basis. That would help the Molokai veterans a lot. We need a lot more, but that would help us a lot.

We also need about $3 million to build our veterans center.

[Laughter and applause.]

Senator AKAKA. Mahalo. Mahalo, Larry.

Dr. Kekahuna, thank you for providing us with that demonstration of what a blinded veteran endures to complete simple tasks. Can you tell us what you mean exactly by "low vision services"? What does that encompass?

Dr. KEKAHUNA. Low vision, in the VA vernacular, is people that are not legally blind or blind. But when administering the test for the low vision test like I go through, they use a lot of different types of equipment, equipment that's needed here in the VA in Honolulu, that tests your eyes to see what your peripheral vision will be and what your central vision will be. It lets, you look deep into the depths of your eyes and how clearly you can see.

I believe that with the equipment and with trained personnel, especially at the medical doctor's level, an MD, that, you know, it would really help the veterans here.

Senator AKAKA. Thank you. Mahalo.

Mr. Helm, Larry, I noted in your testimony that you expressed the need for support of young returning war veterans. Can you tell us what can be done to ease their transition from the military to civilian life?

But before you answer that, let me tell you that one day I was on Maui, and this would have been last year, and there was a Hawaiian father who was hanging around outside. And so when I was ready to leave, he was in a parking lot waiting for me. And he wanted to talk to me.

And he told me the story. He said, you know, my son, before he joined the Army, he used to go surfing. He used to go with his friends. He was always out of the house. And he said, he joined up. He got sent to Iraq when the Iraq War broke out. He served in that war. And then following that, he retired and came home.

And he told me, he said, what can you do to help my son? He said, I can't even get him to surf. He said, he comes home and he sits in the house. And, he said, that's not like him. So he told me, visit with your friends. He said, [inaudible]. And for, I don't know how many months since then, and he saw me, he said, what can I do with my boy? You know, [inaudible].

And I thought I'd mention that. And I don't know what we ought to say. Mahalo.

Mr. HELM. Yes, Senator. Unfortunately, that's the cost of war, that returning young veterans, you're going to have a lot of these kind of situations going on. But there is an asset in every community in this country that if it was to be malama'd or massaged or used, it's the combat veteran that is disabled in every place.

If the VA could put these young guys in touch with these veteran organizations or combat veterans, they know the talk. They know the walk. They've been there, done that, and they could be of great help to these young veterans. That should be one way, besides the VA and the mental health department.

Of course, you need more people in mental health because we have a lot of these young guys coming back. But that's an asset that this country has, is the Vietnam veteran, combat vets, you know, the Korean vets, have been there, have done that, know how to respond to these guys and can help them.

Senator AKAKA. Mahalo, Larry.

Rogelio Evangelista, in your testimony you mentioned that although some veterans live on limited financial support, VA continues to explore raising the co-payments for drugs prescribed for non-service-connected patients. You also mentioned that these same veterans may have limited resources because of physical or mental conditions that can be attributed to their service.

Can you please elaborate on that?

Mr. EVANGELISTA. Well, Senator, in regards to that, I have seen a lot of veterans suffering from PTSD. And because of their physical and mental condition, they work menial jobs and they don't last in those jobs long enough to be fruitful and so forth. So they end up getting laid off. They end up getting in trouble.

And the part is, if we can look at the veteran himself and see how we can retrain him to get, you know, a different type of profession other than just the low, menial type of jobs like, for example, a computer expert, that part, it's something that we can get in regards to this mentality, use it, and we can be accepted back into society by that aspect.

Senator AKAKA. Thank you. Mahalo. Thank you very much.

Before I say mahalo nui loa to this panel, I want to thank all the veterans from Molokai, from Lanai, and of course from Maui, those who traveled here today. It's not very easy—to wake up, to catch the ferry, it's not easy, and I thank you all for making such an effort to get here to testify and to be part of this hearing.

So mahalo nui loa, and I'll turn it over to the Chairman.

Chairman CRAIG. Well, gentlemen, thank you again for your testimony. It's great [inaudible]. Thank you. We'll excuse this panel, and ask our second and last panel to come forward, please. Thank you very much.

[Applause.]

Chairman CRAIG. All right. Let's get started with the second panel. I'm very pleased today that we have—I suspect it's a first on this island—the Under Secretary for Health, Department of Veterans Affairs. This gentleman that I am about to introduce is in charge. It doesn't mean you can blame him for everything. But you can blame him for most. How's that?

[Laughter.]

Chairman CRAIG. Let me introduce to you the Honorable Jonathan A. Perlin, MD, PhD, Under Secretary for Veterans Affairs. He is accompanied by Dr. Robert Wiebe, VA Network Director, VISN 21, Sierra Pacific Network. That's the greater region of the Pacific area. Dr. James Hastings, Director of VA Pacific Islands Health Care Services; and Dr. Steven MacBride, Chief of Staff, Honolulu VA Hospital.

So all four are doctors. I don't know whether that's good or bad.

[Laughter.]

Chairman CRAIG. I suspect in this business it's good. If they were all four lawyers——

[Laughter.]

Chairman CRAIG. I'll let that speak for itself. Somebody said, "We'd be here longer." That's a reasonable observation.

Well, anyway, we thank these gentlemen very much for accompanying us and being with us today. Sitting and listening to your concerns is extremely important for those who make the system work as well as it does, both from the Washington level or from the regional or area level. So we thank you all for being here, and I'll turn the testimony over to Dr. Perlin.

Doctor.

[Applause.]

STATEMENT OF THE HONORABLE JONATHAN A. PERLIN, MD, PhD, UNDER SECRETARY FOR HEALTH, DEPARTMENT OF VETERANS AFFAIRS, ACCOMPANIED BY ROBERT WIEBE, MD, VA NETWORK DIRECTOR, VISN 21, SIERRA PACIFIC NETWORK; JAMES HASTINGS, MD, DIRECTOR, VA PACIFIC ISLANDS HEALTH CARE SYSTEM; AND STEVEN A. MacBRIDE, MD, CHIEF OF STAFF, VA PACIFIC ISLANDS HEALTH CARE SYSTEM

Dr. PERLIN. Aloha, Chairman Craig, Senator Akaka. Mahalo nui loa for the opportunity to be here with you all today to provide testimony, and especially for the opportunity to hear from the men and women of this great State and the veterans who do in fact use

VA for what Chairman Craig and you, with your fine support and advocacy, have helped to shape as the world's best healthcare.

I appreciate the opportunity to hear about ways in which we can improve healthcare here in Maui and on Lanai and on Molokai. And I think today that you will be pleased to hear of a number of improvements that will in fact go a long way toward addressing some of the issues that have been brought to our attention.

It doesn't mean that we'll solve all issues today, but it does mean that I think you will be very pleased to hear some of the progress, and I think I heard in your testimony what I experienced this morning when I had the great honor and privilege of visiting the CBOC here at Maui.

What I saw this morning were a team of dedicated healthcare professionals, staff also, from the Veterans Benefits Administration who not only were technically excellent in their delivery of healthcare services, but in fact, were absolutely passionate and compassionate and really creative in the delivery of those services to individuals that they felt were nothing less than family, part of the community.

There were two doctors, a nurse practitioner. Everyone knows the psychologist, Captain McNamara. In fact, a psychiatrist will soon be joining the team who's also well-known to the residents and veterans of Maui and Molokai and Lanai, Dr. Springer.

And so in that vein, sir, I'm very pleased to be able to report that the VA finds exceptional service to veterans of Maui County through our VA Pacific healthcare system, which is part of the Sierra Pacific Network, one of our 21 Veterans Integrated Service Networks or VISNs.

We're proud to tell you that last year more than 80 percent of our patients at the Maui Outpatient Clinic in fact rated their care as, overall, very good or excellent. We made investments in this clinic 3 years ago, spending more than $200,000 to renovate this clinic into really one of the very nicest.

The clinic staffing complement, as mentioned, includes a full-time primary care physician, a part-time family practice physician. It will include a psychiatrist shortly, the psychologist I mentioned, a nurse practitioner. And we need to extend these services to veterans with specialty care by clinicians who actually rotate to the clinic, such as my colleague, who is not only director of the VA Pacific Islands Healthcare Care System, Dr. James Hastings, but also a cardiologist who is well-known to both the patients and staff, who comes to deliver cardiac care services at this particular clinic.

To further serve the veterans of Maui County, we regularly send VA staff not only from Honolulu, but also as far away as California to bring in the most specialized expertise in all areas. And if veterans services are not available here, then we will make care available in the community, pay for care, in places like Maui Memorial Hospital or in fact Tripler Medical Center as well.

The facts are that last year we spent nearly $3.4 million for non-VA care in the private sector to residents of Maui. I'm also pleased to note that Maui Clinic has—in fact, very shortly—plans for new patients, and it's very rare that patients ever wait more than 30 days for their first appointment.

Senators, the Islands of Molokai and Lanai are also, as all know here, a part of our Maui County service area. And I understand and heard loudly this morning that you've asked us to improve services to those islands. Our staff do visit from Maui, and while we don't operate formal outpatient clinics there, we do provide service to an area which does have a number of veterans.

The island of Molokai, approximately 260 square miles in area, is home to 144 veterans among its population of 649 veterans who use VA for care. We currently send a primary care physician to Molokai once a month, a nurse practitioner once a month, a psychologist twice a month, and we lease space in the community to provide these services.

In addition, we spent more than $250,000 last year to purchase care in the community for eligible veterans living in Molokai at places such as Molokai General Hospital. And we are absolutely thrilled to welcome Dr. Hafermann, a retired Air Force physician, to really be part of the VA community in extending continuity of care on Molokai, supported by what we'll discuss later, I'm sure, increased tele-health services.

I want to thank Senator Akaka for his help in helping to bring Dr. Hafermann to VA as part of our community, and for his support with Chairman Craig of veterans and VA in general. I think it's really important that all here understand the degree of passion and advocacy and courage that you, sir, Senator Akaka and Chairman Craig, show not only for all veterans, but in support of the Department of Veterans Affairs providing services.

VA is working to establish additional tele-health capabilities on Molokai, and has designated our presence there as an outreach clinic. This allows us to establish an electronic link between Molokai and Maui so that electronic health records will also support the clinical care on Molokai.

The island of Lanai is approximately 140 square miles, and VA estimates that the veteran population on the island is 229, of whom 34 veterans use VA for healthcare or used VA for healthcare last year. Similarly, we send a nurse practitioner from the Maui CBOC to Lanai every few months to provide needed primary care services. I believe this can be enhanced in part through care in the community, and last year we spent $35,000 paying for care for veterans in the community, mostly for services through Lanai Community Hospital.

Now, on Lanai, we are not planning to activate a formal community-based outpatient clinic. Instead, we are looking at other options to improve access. We're talking with the Hawaii Health Systems Corporation, the Native Hawaiian Health System, and local providers to potentially establish a federally Qualified Health Center.

Since healthcare is currently limited to residents of Lanai—for example, there are no mental health services on the entire island—we're very excited about the possibilities that this offers to improve healthcare, not just for veterans, but for all residents of the island.

We're also looking at the feasibility of establishing tele-health capabilities on Lanai, and are considering developing contracts with other clinicians to provide care for veterans, much like we're doing on Molokai.

And so in conclusion, with the support of Congress, but in particular with your leadership, Chairman Craig, Ranking Member Akaka, VA is providing unprecedented levels of healthcare services to veterans residing in Maui County, and we look forward to augmenting those with not only new staff such as Dr. Hafermann, but additional tele-health capabilities, and look forward to discussing some of the issues that were raised this morning. Mahalo nui loa.

[Applause.]

[The Prepared statement of Dr. Perlin follows:]

PREPARED STATEMENT OF HON. JONATHAN A. PERLIN, MD, PHD, UNDER SECRETARY FOR HEALTH, DEPARTMENT OF VETERANS AFFAIRS

Mr. Chairman and Members of the Committee, mahalo nui loa for the opportunity to appear before you today to discuss the state of VA care in Hawaii. It is a privilege to be here on Maui—the Valley Isle—to speak and answer questions about issues important to veterans residing in Hawaii.

First, Mr. Chairman, I would like to thank you for your outstanding leadership and advocacy on behalf of our Nation's veterans. During your tenure as Chairman of this Committee, you have clearly demonstrated your commitment to veterans by acting decisively to ensure the needs of veterans are met. In addition, I appreciate your interest in and support of the Department of Veterans Affairs (VA).

I also would like to express my appreciation and respect for Senator Akaka, Ranking Member of this Committee. Along with his colleague, Senator Inouye, Senator Akaka has done so much for the veterans residing in Hawaii and other islands in the Pacific region. As I will highlight later, his vision, guidance and assistance have directly led to an unprecedented level of health care services for veterans, construction of state-of-the-art facilities in Honolulu and remarkable improvements in access to health care services for veterans residing on neighbor islands, including Maui.

Today, I will briefly review the VA Sierra Pacific Network that includes Hawaii and the Pacific region; provide an overview of the VA Pacific Islands Health Care System (VAPIHCS) and the VA clinic here in Maui; highlight issues of particular interest to veterans residing in Maui County, including VA services on the nearby islands of Molokai and Lanai and access to specialty care; and address any questions posed by Members of the Committee.

VA SIERRA PACIFIC NETWORK (VISN 21)

The VA Sierra Pacific Network (Veterans Integrated Service Network [VISN] 21) is one of 21 integrated health care networks in the Veterans Health Administration (VHA). The VA Sierra Pacific Network provides services to veterans residing in Hawaii and the Pacific Basin (including the Philippines, Guam, American Samoa and Commonwealth of the Northern Marianas Islands), northern Nevada and central/northern California. There are an estimated 1.25 million veterans living within the boundaries of the VA Sierra Pacific Network.

The VA Sierra Pacific Network includes six major health care systems based in Honolulu, HI; Palo Alto, CA; San Francisco, CA; Sacramento, CA; Fresno, CA and Reno, NV. Dr. Robert Wiebe serves as director and oversees clinical and administrative operations throughout the Network. In Fiscal Year 2005 (FY05), the Network provided services to 227,000 veterans. There were about 2.8 million clinic stops and 24,000 inpatient admissions. . The cumulative full-time employment equivalents (FTEE) level was 8,200 and the operating budget was about $1.3 billion, which is an increase of $378 million since 2001.

The VA Sierra Pacific Network is remarkable in several ways. In fiscal year 2005, the Network was the only VISN in VHA to meet the performance targets for all six Clinical Interventions that directly address adherence to evidence-based clinical practice. The Network hosts 11 (out of 65) VHA Centers of Excellence—the most in VHA. The VA Sierra Pacific Network also has the highest funded research programs in VHA. Finally, VISN 21 operates one of four Polytrauma units that are dedicated to addressing the clinical needs of the most severely wounded Operation Iraqi Freedom/Operation Enduring Freedom (OIF/OEF) veterans.

VA PACIFIC ISLANDS HEALTH CARE SYSTEM (VAPIHCS)

As noted above, VAPIHCS is one of six major health care systems in VISN 21. VAPIHCS is unique in several important aspects: its vast catchment area covering 2.6 million square-miles (including Hawaii, Guam, American Samoa and Commonwealth of the Northern Marianas); island topography and the challenges to access it creates; richness of the culture of Pacific Islanders; and the ethnic diversity of patients and staff. In fiscal year 2005, there were an estimated 113,000 veterans living in Hawaii (9 percent of Network total).

VAPIHCS provides care in six locations: Ambulatory Care Center (ACC) and Center for Aging (CFA) on the campus of the Tripler Army Medical Center (AMC) in Honolulu; and community-based outpatient clinics (CBOCs) in Lihue (Kauai), Kahului (Maui), Kailua-Kona (Hawaii), Hilo (Hawaii) and Agana (Guam). VAPIHCS also sends clinicians and support staff from these locations to provide services on Lanai, Molokai and American Samoa. The inpatient post-traumatic stress disorder (PTSD) unit formerly in Hilo is in the process of relocating to Honolulu. In addition to VAPIHCS, VHA operates five Readjustment Counseling Centers (Vet Centers) in Honolulu, Lihue, Wailuku, Kailua-Kona and Hilo that provide counseling, psychosocial support and outreach.

Dr. James Hastings was recently appointed Director, VAPIHCS. Dr. Hastings has impressive credentials, including tenure as Chair, Department of Medicine, John A. Burns School of Medicine, University of Hawaii, and Commanding General at Walter Reed AMC and Tripler AMC. I am excited about the possibilities that his tenure as Director at VAPIHCS brings.

In fiscal year 2005, VAPIHCS provided services to 18,300 veterans in Hawaii (8 percent of Network total). There were 194,000 clinic stops in Hawaii during fiscal year 2005 (7 percent of Network total), an increase of 36 percent since fiscal year 2000. The cumulative FTEE for the health care system was 478 employees. The budget for VAPIHCS (including General Purpose, Specific Purpose and Medical Care Cost Funds [MCCF]) has increased from $53 million in fiscal year 1999 to $102 million in fiscal year 2005 (about 8 percent of Network total). In addition, VISN 21 provided over $20 million in supplemental funds to VAPIHCS over the past two Fiscal Years to ensure VAPIHCS met its financial obligations.

VAPIHCS provides or contracts for a comprehensive array of health care services. VAPIHCS directly provides primary care, including preventive services and health screenings, and mental health services at all locations. Selected specialty services are also currently provided at the Honolulu campus and to a lesser extent, at CBOCs. VAPIHCS recently hired specialists in gero-psychiatry, gastroenterology, ophthalmology and radiology. VAPIHCS is actively recruiting additional specialists in cardiology, orthopedic surgery and urology. Inpatient long-term care is available at the 60-bed Center for Aging. Inpatient mental health services are provided by VA staff on a 20-bed ward within Tripler AMC and at the 16-bed PTSD Residential Rehabilitation Program (PRRP) that was formerly in Hilo (now relocating to Honolulu). VAPIHCS contracts for care with DoD (at Tripler AMC and Guam Naval Hospital) and community facilities for inpatient medical-surgical care.

The current constellation of VA facilities and services represents a remarkable transformation over the past several years. Previously, the VAPIHCS (formerly known as the VA Medical and Regional Office Center [VAMROC] Honolulu) operated primary care and mental health clinics based in the Prince Kuhio Federal Building in downtown Honolulu and CBOCs on the neighbor islands that were staffed primarily with nurse practitioners. Senator Akaka and his colleagues in Congress approved $83 million in Major Construction funds to build a state-of-the-art ambulatory care center and nursing home care unit on the Tripler AMC campus and these facilities were activated in 2000 and 1997, respectively. VISN 21 allocated nearly $17 million from FY98–FY00 to activate these projects. VISN 21 also provided dedicated funds (e.g., $2 million in fiscal year 2001) to enhance care on the neighbor islands by expanding/renovating clinic space and adding additional staff to ensure there are primary care physicians and psychiatrists at all CBOCs.

MAUI CBOC

VA operates a CBOC, located in Kahului (203 Ho'ohana, Suite 303, Kahului, HI, 96732). In fiscal year 2002, VAPIHCS spent $208,000 to renovate the clinic. The Maui Vet Center is located in nearby Wailuku.

The veterans treated at the Maui CBOC appear to be very satisfied with their care. For example, a Vietnam veteran recently remarked, "I chose VA when I had opportunities to use other health care. My medical care from the Maui CBOC has been superb in every respect. There is genuine concern for my health and well-being and I could not hope for better care." With comments like this, it is not surprising that in fiscal year 2005, VAPIHCS achieved an exceptional level of performance in the national VHA measure of outpatient satisfaction with over 80 percent of patients rating their overall care as "very good" or "excellent."

The Maui CBOC serves an estimated island veteran population in fiscal year 2005 of 10,787. In fiscal year 2005, 2,769 veterans were enrolled for care and 1,464 veterans received care ("users") at the Maui CBOC. The market penetrations for enrollees and "users" are 26 percent and 14 percent, respectively, and compare favorably with rates within VISN 21 and VHA.

The current authorized full-time employment equivalents (FTEE) level is 12.4, including a full-time primary care physician, part-time family practice physician, psychiatrist, psychologist and nurse practitioner. With this staff, the Maui CBOC provides a broad range of primary care and mental health services. In addition, VAPIHCS provides specialty care services at the clinic by sending VA staff from Honolulu and other VA facilities in California. Services provided by clinicians traveling to Maui include cardiology, geriatrics, nephrology, neurology, optometry, orthopedics, rheumatology and urology. If veterans need services not available at the clinic, VAPIHCS arranges and pays for care in the local community (e.g., Maui Memorial Hospital), Honolulu (including Tripler AMC) or VA facilities in California. In fiscal year 2005, VA spent nearly $3.4 million for non-VA care in the private sector (i.e., not including costs at other VA or DoD facilities) for residents of Maui.

In fiscal year 2005, the Maui CBOC recorded 9,135 clinic stops, representing a 41 percent increase from fiscal year 2000 (i.e., 6,499 stops). The clinic has short waiting times for new patients with very few veterans waiting more than 30 days for their first primary care appointment.

SPECIAL ISSUES

The islands of Molokai and Lanai are part of Maui County. Although VA provides limited services on these islands by VA staff visiting from Maui, VA does not operate formal CBOCs in these locations. Veterans and their advocates have asked VA to increase services in these underserved areas.

Molokai. The area of the island of Molokai is approximately 260 square miles. VA estimates the veteran population to be 649. In fiscal year 2005, 202 veterans were enrolled for VA care and 144 veterans received VA services. VA currently sends a primary care physician to Molokai once a month, a nurse practitioner once a month and a psychologist twice a month. VA leases space in the community to provide these services. In addition, VA purchased non-VA care in the community (e.g., Molokai General Hospital) for eligible veterans residing in Molokai (e.g., $254 thousand in fiscal year 2005). Veterans residing in Molokai also are seen at DoD and VA facilities in other locations.

In fiscal year 2005, VHA formally designated the VA presence in Maui as an outreach clinic. This allowed VAPIHCS to establish an electronic link between the outreach clinic in Molokai and the Maui CBOC so that the VA electronic medical record can be used in Molokai. At present, due to the relatively small number of veterans residing in Molokai, VA does not plan to establish a formal CBOC in Molokai. However, VA does plan to improve access to health care services on the island.

Based on information provided by Senator Akaka and his staff, VA has identified a former Air Force physician (i.e., Dr. Hafermann) who resides in Molokai and is interested in providing medical care to veterans on a part-time basis. VAPIHCS recently credentialed and privileged this physician and is working with him to establish a regular clinic schedule in early 2006. VA is also working to establish telehealth capabilities from Molokai. VA will place an order for telehealth equipment and is working to identify the location for the telehealth activities. VA will also explore the possibility of sharing telehealth capabilities with non-VA providers in exchange for local services for veterans.

Lanai. The island of Lanai is approximately 140 square-miles. VA estimates the veteran population to be 229. In fiscal year 2005, 57 veterans were enrolled for VA care and 34 veterans received VA services. VA currently sends a nurse practitioner from the Maui CBOC to Lanai every couple of months to provide needed primary care services. In addition, VA purchased non-VA care in the community (e.g., Lanai Community Hospital) for eligible veterans residing in Lanai (e.g., $35 thousand in fiscal year 2005). Veterans residing in Lanai also are seen at DoD and VA facilities in other locations.

Due to the small number of veterans residing in Lanai, VA does not plan to activate a formal CBOC. Instead, VA is exploring other options to improve access. VA is talking with the Hawaii Health Systems Corporation (HHSC), Native Hawaiian Health System and local providers (i.e., Straub Clinic) to potentially establish a federally Qualified Health Center (FQHC). Since health care is limited to all residents of Lanai (e.g., there are no mental health services in Lanai), a FQHC offers exciting possibilities. VA is also exploring the feasibility of establishing telehealth capabilities in Lanai. Finally, VA will also consider establishing a contract with local clinicians to provide care for veterans, based on the availability of resources and local interest.

Specialty services. The size of the veteran population and number of VA patients limit the feasibility of having a large cadre of medical and surgical specialists based in the Maui CBOC. Nonetheless, VA recognizes that some veterans in Maui County have needs that go beyond primary care and mental health. As I noted earlier, VA sends specialists from Honolulu and California to the clinic on a regular basis. Services provided by clinicians traveling to Maui include cardiology, geriatrics, nephrology, neurology, optometry, orthopedics, rheumatology and urology. VAPIHCS also refers patients to the local community for care at VA expense (when eligibility criteria are met) and transports (also at VA expense when eligibility criteria are met) patients to the VA facility in Honolulu.

VAPIHCS is utilizing telehealth technology to expand access to specialty care (e.g., dermatology). VAPIHCS estimates that telehealth services are provided more than 15 hours per week at the Maui CBOC. As additional specialists are hired at the VA facility based in Honolulu, these clinicians will be able to travel to Maui County and further utilize telehealth technologies. For the past several years, veterans in Maui have been invited to participate in research studies designed to test if telehealth could be used effectively to extend mental health services (e.g., treatment for PTSD) to a culturally diverse population. The willingness of Maui veterans to participate reflects their trust in VAPIHCS, Maui Vet Center and VHA National Center for PTSD.

As noted before, VAPIHCS staff occasionally refers patients to VA facilities in California. Access to other VA facilities was especially important to a veteran who wrote, "The veteran's health center in Kona [Kailua-Kona CBOC] has not only helped me get my prescription drugs at a lower cost, but last year they helped me go to the Western Blind Rehabilitation Center in Palo Alto to learn how to cope with my blindness. For the first time in many years, I have confidence to do things I never thought I could do without sight."

CONCLUSION

In summary, with the support of Senator Akaka and other Members of Congress, VA is providing an unprecedented level of health care services to veterans residing in Hawaii and the Pacific Region. VA now has state-of-the-art facilities and enhanced services in Honolulu, as well as robust staffing on the neighbor islands and has expanded or renovated clinics in many locations. VA is bringing more specialists on board and preparing for the newest generation of veterans-those who bravely served in southwest Asia.

VAPIHCS still faces several challenges, in part due to the topography of its catchment area. VAPIHCS will meet these challenges by utilizing telehealth technologies, sharing specialists, developing new delivery models and opening new clinics as demographics suggest and resources allow. I am proud of the improvements in VA services in Hawaii, but recognize that our job is not done.

Again, Mr. Chairman and other Members of the Committee, mahalo nui loa for the opportunity to testify at this hearing. I would be delighted to address any questions you may have for me or other members of the panel.

Chairman CRAIG. Thank you very much, Dr. Perlin. You mentioned in your testimony that VA does send a primary care physician and a nurse practitioner to Molokai once per month, and a psychologist to the island twice per month, to provide service to veterans who reside there.

What kind of service does the traveling staff generally provide? Is there an advance schedule of their travel published so that all veterans on the island know of the staff's impending arrival?

Dr. PERLIN. Thank you, Chairman Craig, for the question. In fact, I asked that question this morning when we had the chance to visit the Maui CBOC. In fact, the nurse practitioner and the primary care physician provide just that, general medical care. They make appropriate referrals where that is necessary.

Captain McNamara, the psychologist, provides individual psychotherapy and support services, outreach counseling, across the range of mental health diagnoses. Again, she also makes appropriate referrals. I know, as was alluded to here, she also looks forward to

Dr. Springer coming back to the Maui CBOC to be part of the mental health team.

We realize that that is one way of extending our outreach, is to provide the services with physicians, psychologists, who travel. But we also look forward to extending the reach of telehealth as one of the important ways to help provide additional support.

We do publish a schedule annually of the times that the medical team is there. But one of the other things that we also discussed that the clinic does is that they send a letter individually to each patient to just reaffirm particular appointment times.

Chairman CRAIG. Well, thank you. One of the gentlemen who testified on the first panel mentioned that there were some difficulties experienced by some of his friends in obtaining quick and accurate travel reimbursement from VA for his visit to—I think this was to Honolulu for services.

Can you or someone else on the panel here give me an idea of what the process of beneficiary travel reimbursement is like, and what turnaround time there is on these claims?

Dr. PERLIN. Let me just note that, in fact, the backlog of claims has been worked down so that once the claim is received, it should be less than 30 days. But let me ask Dr. MacBride to elaborate on the current process.

Dr. MACBRIDE. Thank you very much. Thank you, Dr. Perlin.

Patients who have had authorization for travel then have the opportunity to submit travel claims for reimbursement. Typically, we receive those requests for reimbursement anywhere from 6 to 8 weeks after the travel has occurred, sometimes sooner.

From that point on, it takes us about 30 days in processing. As Dr. Perlin mentioned, we did have a backlog for a while in our claims processing. So once we are in receipt of completed claim with a receipt, we are able to refund the veteran within 30 days.

Chairman CRAIG. Dr. MacBride, if you would explain to me, and maybe to the audience, what designates—I believe you used the word certified travel—or authorized travel. Yes. How is that established?

Dr. MACBRIDE. Well, travel for veterans that is going to be reimbursed by the VA is authorized ahead of time. Typically, our travel benefits include travel for service-connected conditions.

Chairman CRAIG. So in other words, that's known in advance by the veteran who's traveling to seek services, whether he or she has been authorized——

Dr. MACBRIDE. That's correct.

Chairman T4raig [Continuing]. To receive reimbursement?

Dr. MACBRIDE. That's correct, sir.

Chairman CRAIG. Dr. Perlin, you mentioned in your testimony that VA purchased approximately $250,000 worth of care and services from Molokai General Hospital for veterans residing there.

What criteria governs the decision to purchase care locally on the island as opposed to having veterans travel to other places for care, and are those standards for Hawaii any different than any of the other States?

Dr. PERLIN. Mr. Chairman, that is a great question. And in fact, there's absolutely no difference in the way that one makes a purchase or provides service decision or [inaudible] decision. It comes down to this. If the veteran has an emergency situation, and those are emergencies to a reasonable person—someone who has chest pain—then we buy those services.

You know, when there is some time there, we really do appreciate when the veteran calls to make sure that we can coordinate services as well as possible. These are small communities. Doctors and nurses and psychologists and others know each other. So that if there's an urgent situation or emergency, we will purchase those services.

We won't purchase the services, A, if they're not available because they're not available of the island of Molokai, for example, itself; or when in fact we know that it's not an emergency or urgent situation, and we not only have the services, but by virtue of the electronic health record and the continuity and quality that both you and Senator Akaka alluded to, we can provide those services within VA. So emergency or urgent, we purchase otherwise services that we would provide ourselves.

Senator AKAKA. Dr. Hastings and Dr. MacBride, as you know, last year I introduced legislation to formalize what VA is already doing on Molokai and to increase access to VA care.

I understand that VA sent a team to Molokai to review certain options. Will you please describe those options? Have there been any attempts to coordinate with Mr. Helm's group, Molokai Veterans Caring for Veterans, as they have identified land to build a center for veterans on the island that could potentially house a part-time clinic or, at the very least, space to house tele-ealth equipment? Please make your remarks on this.

Dr. HASTINGS. Senator, Dr. MacBride is part of that group. So I've asked him to respond to your question.

Senator AKAKA. Dr. MacBride?

Dr. MACBRIDE. Thank you, Dr. Hastings. Thank you, Senator Akaka. I want to thank also Mr. Larry Helm and Mr. Manny Garcia and Dr. Dave Hafermann and several other Molokai veterans who not only joined us on that day, but provided us with some very interesting insights into care and conditions on Molokai that helped us enormously.

As was mentioned earlier, for a number of years now staff from the Maui CBOC have been traveling to Molokai to provide services in a rural health clinic located on the grounds of Molokai General Hospital. I think that it's worth mentioning—some of them haven't been mentioned today—a person who really went forward first was Kathy Haas, CNS who at the time was our nurse practitioner in the CBOC in Maui and now coordinates the management of all of our CBOCS.

[Applause.]

Dr. MACBRIDE. And then in addition, we have heard so many nice things said about Kathy McNamara, Dr. Jim Santoro, Rita Webb, and previously, Dr. Richard Rose, the psychiatrist.

There on Molokai, what we did in fiscal year 2005, as Dr. Perlin testified, was to designate our presence at the Rural Health Clinic as an outreach of the Maui CBOC, an outreach clinic. With that official designation in VA, it allowed us to provide the electronic links to establish connectivity to the VA electronic patient record.

This is extremely important because, in fact, this is really the lifeblood of our care, to be able to have the electronic record throughout VA so that the record is present wherever veterans travel. Veterans don't travel with the record. With that established, we have now gone forward, and Dr. Dave Hafermann, who was introduced earlier, a retired Air Force internist/pulmonologist—that's a lung specialist—will begin seeing veteran patients in the Rural Health Clinic using our electronic record in February of this year.

In addition, VA, with its partnerships with Queen's Medical Center and the administration of Molokai General Hospital, will be using tele-health equipment that is in existence at the Molokai General Hospital. Further, we will augmenting that equipment with VA tele-health equipment.

Now, it's fortunate that the Molokai General Hospital is linked to the State Tele-health Access Network, the STAN. That allows us to have the broadband that is necessary to do tele-health transmissions.

We were fortunate that day to review several other options and availabilities, and meet several of the physicians on the island. There is a federally Qualified Health Center in Kaunakakai, and there is Hui Malama with the Native Hawaiian Health Care System. We plan to work more closely with the Native Hawaiian Health Care System because they are expert at providing education for chronic diseases. We, in addition, are expert at providing tele-mental health for mental health services in general.

So, in addition to our traveling people to Molokai, we intend to work with our new physician, Dr. Hafermann, physicians in the community hopefully by contract, and to augment services using telehealth.

I also want to thank Larry Helms and Manny Garcia and Dr. Dave Hafermann for their service to veterans, and not only through the insights they provided to VA leadership, but also in showing us their plans for the veterans center. Our mission, of course, is to provide healthcare services to the 144 veterans who Dr. Perlin mentioned have enrolled for care with us and are actively receiving VA services. We look forward to working closely with Mr. Helm and Mr. Garcia and the Koa Kahiko to explore and establish the best possible options for enhanced care for Molokai's veterans.

Senator AKAKA. Thank you very much for that response, Dr. MacBride.

Dr. Perlin, your testimony indicates that VA does not plan to activate a formal clinic on Lanai. Can you explain some other ways that VA can improve access to care for veterans on Lanai? I am especially interested in hearing more about a federally Qualified Health Center that could benefit all veterans on Lanai.

Dr. PERLIN. Thank you, Senator Akaka, for that question. As with Molokai, the ability to improve services for the residents of that island occurs through more regularly scheduled visits and additional visits of staff, better coordination with the local providers in the community, and the use of telehealth, which we're exploring.

All that said, I'm very excited, as well of its acceptance for a federally Qualified Health Center, and I would again ask to turn the microphone back to Dr. MacBride to elaborate on that discussion.

Dr. MACBRIDE. Well, thank you, Dr. Perlin. And before I forget, I would like to take the opportunity to thank you, Senator Craig, for coming all the way out to Hawaii in January, and Senator Akaka, for your remarkable leadership and assistance here with veterans here and the VA.

The VA is very fortunate again on the island of Lanai to have discovered recently that we have the opportunity to work together with partners and friends. Mr. Tom Driskill, who testified yesterday in Kauai and who is the CEO for the Hawaii Health Systems Corporation, and Mr. Ray Vera from Straub Clinic and Hospital, recently discussed with us the opportunity to collaborate together.

On Lanai, the hospital is administered by Hawaii Health Systems Corporation, and they have the outpatient building in which Straub Clinic houses two physicians who practice medicine and also do emergency services at the hospital.

There is a plan, with VA in collaboration, to apply for a federally Qualified Health Clinic and to add much-needed women's services to the island—and I think Mr. Obado testified to the importance of having services for women as well—and also to partner with Native Hawaiian Health Care System in their remarkable ability to provide education for chronic diseases.

We very much want to partner with these individuals amenities. We want to be able work with physicians onsite who can see our VA patients and take care of VA patients in the event of an emergency. But we also want to augment mental health services in which VA is so outstanding. So we intend to provide tele-mental health services for patients of this consortium with whom we work. In addition, our partners have spoken with us about the possibility of supplementing some of the specialty care, and we will study that as well.

Senator AKAKA. Thank you very much for your response, Dr. MacBride.

Dr. Wiebe, I have concerns about the Maui clinic and other clinics around Hawaii restricting specific healthcare services such as home care, based upon disabilities status rather than clinical need. I am glad that VA is reviewing this situation. I know they are.

I need a commitment from you that when these restrictions are lifted, that new dollars will flow from the network to Hawaii to cover these costs. But we'd like to hear your thoughts about this.

Dr. WIEBE. Thank you, Senator Akaka. As you know, the Pacific Islands Health Care System is one of six healthcare systems that comprise the VA Sierra Pacific Network. One of my responsibilities as network director is to make an allocation to each facility at the beginning of each fiscal year.

Since I have been network director and have had the privilege of doing so since 1998, budget at the VA Pacific Island Health Care System has increased from approximately $53 million to, last year, about $105 million. The portion of that budget that is allocated by my office to Hawaii, has increased over this period of time by 85 percent, while the network budget, as a whole, has increased about 70 percent.

I expect that the budget here in Hawaii for fiscal year 2006—that allocation has not been made yet—that the allocation will be higher than the previous year. In general, we do not allocate money for individual programs, but instead rely on each individual medical center and healthcare system to make those choices based upon what they know the local conditions and the local needs to be.

You're absolutely correct in that we were, here, incorrectly and inappropriately restricting care. That since has been corrected, and I fully expect that additional resources will be spent on non-institutional care specifically in the home healthcare programs.

Senator AKAKA. Thank you very much, Dr. Wiebe, for your response.

Dr. Perlin, vision impairment, as you heard from Dr. Kekahuna, services provided veterans are below par in Hawaii, and he compared some services he received on the mainland.

What can be done to improve this situation?

Dr. PERLIN. Well, thank you, Senator Akaka, for that question on care for veterans with blindness or low vision. I need to tell you that this is not a theoretical question for me. My grandfather was a blinded veteran, and something I feel very passionately about. This is also not the first opportunity that I've had the privilege of meeting Dr. Kekahuna or some of his colleagues.

I think the opportunities to improve care here in Hawaii are not significantly different than some of the opportunities to advance for the care for veterans with blindness and low vision. There are really two things that I think we need to think about in caring for veterans with blindness or low vision.

First is the proximity, but the second is the mode in which the veteran acquired blindness. The veteran who experienced the immediate, traumatic loss of vision is one circumstance. The other circumstance is one that's becoming all too prevalent today: Older veterans, or even some veterans who aren't all that old, who have the ravages of diabetes or macular degeneration.

And in fact, for the veteran who's had a sudden and catastrophic loss of vision, a very intensive inpatient setting which has a great deal of experience, such as in a Blind Rehab Center, is really the best way to reorient them to higher function, given the trauma of recent blindness.

I'm pleased that Dr. Kekahuna had such a good experience at the Western Blind Rehabilitation Center, which is one of 10 national referral centers for veterans that are scattered around the country. We just opened a brand-new Blind Rehab Center at Hines where Dr. Kekahuna has also experienced their care. This is a shining example of the promise of the Cares program and the best we can offer veterans. It is a premier facility anywhere in the world.

That doesn't answer the mail, though, for the veteran who has the gradual loss of vision and needs some support in his or her community. In fact, Ms. Cynthia Yosuda is dual-hatted right now. She is the visual impairment coordinator, and she in fact needs to be given more time to provide services and outreach.

This is one of the areas where I think we can improve care here in Hawaii, which is to provide that dedicated time and those important services. I've become aware that there are some equipment needs that are actually fairly modest, and we can provide that as well.

The optometrists do travel, not only to Maui, but Kona and Hilo and Kauai as well. And we do hope to coordinate with the wonderful program that is here in the State that provides services for all residents of the State. But that's not enough. We're also hiring an ophthalmologist who will begin to make rounds, and I'm pleased to report that that individual will be part of the team here in VA Pacific Islands Health Care Systems in 60 days.

Finally, sir, I think one of the best ways to address blindness is to prevent it. I couldn't be more proud of the high-quality care provided by VA in terms of treating diabetes so well and preventing the really horrific complications, such as loss of vision.

Senator AKAKA. Thank you very much, Dr. Perlin, for that response. And I noted in your testimony that VA is working to establish telehealth capabilities on Molokai. Do you have an idea about the timeframe on that?

Dr. PERLIN. We look forward to seeing the telehealth in operation in April. And I'm also pleased to report that VISN 21 and the VA Pacific Islands Healthcare System applied for some funding for telehealth and its support of tele-mental health—and I'm pleased to share a little bit before the announcement, but I want to thank Chairman Craig and Senator Akaka for their support of the mental health initiatives to make this possible—$200,000 to support personnel to operate that equipment in such areas as tele-mental health.

Senator AKAKA. Thank you. I have two more questions, Dr. Perlin.

VA in Hawaii falls under the Sierra Pacific Health Care Network, which includes some very large tertiary facilities in California. Given the competing demands for resources, how do you believe VA Hawaii is faring?

Dr. PERLIN. Well, Senator, I think Dr. Wiebe mentioned that the budgets for the VA Pacific Islands Health Care System increased from $53 million to nearly $105 million over this last 5-year period, roughly doubling. And so it's fairly clear to me that Dr. Wiebe, in making allocation decisions, understands and appreciates the needs for services here in Hawaii and neighbor islands.

I think the budget is good. As both you and Chairman Craig and Secretary Nicholson challenge us, our goal is to make sure that those resources go as far as possible in treating as many veterans as possible, as well as possible.

Senator AKAKA. Thank you. And my final question is one about long-term care needs. Testimony given at yesterday's hearing on Kauai pointed to the significant gaps in long-term care services provided to Hawaii's veterans due to the geography of our State.

What is the VA doing to meet long-term care needs on Maui and throughout all of Hawaii, both in terms of nursing home care and home-based care?

Dr. PERLIN. We appreciate the opportunity to discuss the long-term care. And clearly there are here some veterans who are not safe or don't have social support and need institutional long-term care.

I recall your support and that of this Committee for building the Center for Aging on the Tripler campus, and it's really a remarkable institution. It provides care for up to 60 veterans. And I know that it's been running very full, 56 veterans on average.

I'm very, very excited, again, about the leadership that's been shown in the State of Hawaii to build the new State Veterans Home in Hilo. This is a very exciting proposition. It's a partnership with the State. VA provides two-thirds of the funding for up to $20 million, and we look forward to this facility opening in the spring of 2007, again providing 95 additional beds.

VA contracts for care in a couple of other community nursing homes. We do have some challenges in terms of the institutional care in that any of facilities either don't meet VA's life safety standards, which we consider absolutely critical, or they haven't been willing to contract with us.

We really hope to get Dr. Michael Carrithers, who was here yesterday and is the Associate Chief of Staff of the Pacific Islands Health Care Systems for Geriatric and Extended Care, together with Mr. Driskill, to see what sorts of discussions might bear.

Turning to the non-institutional care, this is really such an important area. It's an area where we've had to preserve not only community relationships but, as in the case of so many World War II veterans, spousal relationships of 50 or 60 years.

The use of technologies that allow us to make sure that the veteran is doing OK, that their breathing is OK, that their weight is OK, that their blood sugar is OK, that they're taking their medicines, that they're not hungry, are technologies that are not science fiction. They're technologies that we use today.

They're technologies that preserve that spousal and community relationship under technologies which also extend the dollars. And I'm very proud of the tremendous increases that are being shown here in Hawaii, which not only offer all of the social advantages, but also transcend and get beyond the barrier of that great ocean that separates the islands.

Senator AKAKA. Thank you so much for your response. I want to especially thank Dr. Hastings and Dr. MacBride for responding to my repeated, really repeated requests for addressing access to care, and those issues on Maui and on Molokai and Lanai. I really am happy to have learned of your efforts to include access to care for rural veterans as well.

I appreciate Dr. Perlin's and Dr. Wiebe's response to these needs as well. I also thank Cathy Haas and Dr. McNamara for what you do every day to help the veterans of Maui County. And I want to thank this panel very much for coming to Hawaii and responding as you have to our questions here. That without question will make a huge difference for all veterans in Hawaii.

I also want to remind you that we have a table in the back of the room where we have staff, both from the VA, as well as our staff, who are there to take any questions or concerns that you may have. Remember that if you're wanting to testify and we don't have it on the agenda, you are welcome to give us a statement or arrange to give a statement to us. And we'll be glad to direct it.

So again, I want to say thank you so much to this distinguished panel that's before us. Also, before I quit here, I want to say mahalo nui loa to Lupe Wissel, who sits on this side of the Chairman, and to Noe Kalipi, who sits on this side, on my side. I also want to thank the Committee staff, Kim Lipsky, Dahlia Melendrez, and Alex Sardegna, who organized this morning's hearing. Thank you so much because it really went well.

And mahalo nui loa for making this a great hearing, Mr. Chairman.

Chairman CRAIG. Well, Danny, thank you very much.

Ladies and gentlemen, my fellow citizens, I am here today and the Committee is here today because of Danny Akaka. He is a gentleman and a soft-spoken person, but one of the loudest advocates you have in Washington, DC.

[Applause.]

Chairman CRAIG. And you watched a classic case this morning of Senator Akaka working with this panel to get them to assure you and him that the services he has consistently requested for you are being looked at and/or are en route toward being supplied. That role he plays on behalf of all of you in the State of Hawaii is a very active one, and I congratulate Danny for his advocacy.

Let me also mention one of you in your testimony of the first panel. You referred to him as a Senator. He is not. He is a Congressman, Congressman Buyer, who is Chairman of the Veterans Affairs Committee in the House. He's been in a bit of controversy of late in discussing how he would handle what had been traditional hearings by the service organizations who come to Washington annually to advocate on your behalf, but also to examine the budgets as proposed by the administrations and the Veterans Administration itself as it relates to its adequacy.

He and I disagree as to how those hearings ought to be held. Please understand me very directly: All veterans service organizations will be heard. We will hold those hearings on the Senate side. Other hearings will be held on the House side. But rest assured, all veterans service organizations who come to Washington to testify before the appropriate authorizing Committee—that's this Committee—will be heard in complete forum as to the record they want to build.

[Applause.]

Chairman CRAIG. Let me also thank this panel, Dr. Perlin and his associates, for being here, for the work they do. I've had the privilege of getting to know these gentlemen, work very closely with Dr. Perlin and of course Robert Wiebe, and I'm getting to know these other gentlemen. And they live their profession on a day-to-day basis. They are without question your greatest advocates.

While there may be times when they make tough choices, that's also their job as it relates to how resources get allocated and where resources go. They live with you on a day-to-day basis. They are committed as no other professionals I have ever met as to the services they provide and the responsibilities they've undertaken with the titles of the positions that they hold. I honor them for that. They should be recognized for that quality of work.

Let me also recognize, as Danny did, Lupe Whistle, who's the staff director for the Veterans' Affairs Committee to my immediate right; Billy Cahill in the back, an associate who, between us all, keep these folks on their toes; because the relationship of Government is a lot of oversight and checks and balances. That's the character of our system and why it works, frankly, as well as it does.

The administrative side, the legislative side, the policymaking side, the budget-shaping side. That's Danny's responsibility. That's my responsibility. The administrative side is to take that policy and the resources and bring it to the ground to provide the services for us to oversight and to view and to correct or adjust as time goes on and the situations occur, and as you react to us, as you should in a representative republic, in the way you have with your presence here today.

We thank you all very much for coming out and spending your morning and early afternoon with us. And again, Danny, let me thank you for inviting me and the Committee to your great State.

[Applause.]

Senator AKAKA. Mahalo. Mahalo nui loa, Mr. Chairman. Larry and I, as you can tell, work very well together. And many of our successes in the Committee are due to him. And so he has done well for the veterans across the country.

But I want to particularly thank him for sacrificing the few days that he has to come to Hawaii and join us with this hearing. He has made a huge difference. And I want to thank him for his generous remarks and wish him a safe trip, and his staff also, when they finally go back to Washington, DC. Larry, I can't thank you enough for helping us out here. Mahalo.

[Applause.]

Chairman CRAIG. Thank you. The Committee will stand adjourned.

[Whereupon, at 12:28 p.m., the Committee was adjourned.]

A P P E N D I X 1

PREPARED STATEMENT OF PATRICIA ABSHER ROSS ON BEHALF OF HER HUSBAND JOHN WILLIAM ROSS, JR., LCDR, USN, RET.

I, Patricia Ross, am a Veteran of the United States Cadet Nurse Corps, sworn into service March, 1944. I received tuition, maintenance, textbooks, Summer and Winter uniforms and stipends, and signed to stay in essential nursing until the war crisis was over. I was released from that commitment in March, 1947, the nursing shortage declared over.

We are registered and included in the Women Veterans' Memorial, Arlington National Cemetery, Washington D.C., the only Congressionally mandated memorial to honor all military women-all wars—all grades—all periods of time from the Revolutionary War to present day and beyond. It is with that service background that I rise to speak-up for my husband, John Ross, and thank you for allowing me the opportunity and honor to do so.

Specifically, I would like to address the issue of the inequity of access to care for the many underserved veterans needing care, in Maui County so they can be supported and be with family and friends, at a critical, frightening, stressful time in their lives.

John has numerous health problems that require Specialists' care and monitoring. We have chosen to pay for Kaiser Permanente Senior Advantage program and use them as our primary care. Because of moderately severe Dementia and being blind, John must stay in familiar surroundings to avoid panic and air travel is not for him. What we seek from the Veterans Health Care System, is help with expenses for Intermediate Day Care and Long-term Care, when it will be needed at home, here on the Island of Maui, where we have been for 29 years.

Medical expenses have been very high this year, with needing to have full time care for John' while his wife was hospitalized with four cardiac surgeries, (February to mid-July). John cannot be left alone. This was an unplanned expense for an exhausted wife, Caregiver!

Nearly 300, Disabled Veterans in Maui County face similar problems.

BRIEF HISTORY

John entered service in the U.S. Navy on March 31, 1941 and was honorably discharged on July 31, 1961. He served in the Navy as a career Engineering Officer (EDO) for over 20 years. He was classified as 100 percent, service-connected disabled effective February 26, 2002, based on diagnosed Asbestosis some years ago, as John developed a malignant lesion in his lung.

Cause	Problem	Medical Monitoring
Ship repair, inspection, construction, mothballing constant exposure to asbestos.	Lung cancer	Pulmonary specialist
Dry-docked radioactive Ships at SFNaval Shipyard from atomic tests at Bikini Atoll, 1948.	Skin Cancers, colon cancer	Dermatologist Surgeon/Oncologist
Numerous head injuries Normal Pressure Starting with 2 falls down Hydrocephalus Darkened submarine Hatches.	Normal pressure, hydrocephalus	Neurologist to monitor shunt placed in brain.
Knee deterioration × 2	Knee Replacements (2)	Orthopedic checks
Vision: Aging	Blindness due to Ophthalmologist, Q2mos.	Ophthalmologist, checks
Prostate problems	Elevated psa (28)	Urologist

(41)

The cost for the medical care was covered by the Kaiser Insurance we have held for many years and will keep as our Primary Care.

DIFFICULTIES ENCOUNTERED WITH MAUI VETERANS HEALTH CARE

Full access for Veterans to have VA Health Care on Maui, Lanai and Molokai, and provisions for intermediate and long term care, at home or in facilities ON IS-LAND does not exist. Numerous agencies and qualified medical personnel are present and could provide much of the care if the VA would contract with them.

John's greatest fear expressed to the VA Gerontologists on 12/15/05, was what would happen to him if something happened to his wife, first! The doctors assured him that he would be taken care of, but in HONOLULU.

It is hard to accept that John would be sent off island, away from his home, friends, and familiar surroundings to a more confusing, unfamiliar place, blind, with mobility problems, worried about his wife of 58 years and no way to keep in touch. He is very frightened.

Reasons given for not contracting on each island vary from:

(1) Excessive pages of redundant paper work required by the VA

(2) The VA is slow in paying and the care facilities cannot carry the debt.

(3) The Veterans are not organized to demand change.

(4) The Veterans are considered a "sub-group" among the numerous health Agencies planning long-term care for Seniors and Disabled.

There re over 13,000 veterans in Maui County.

(5) Permission needed from the VA to participate and there is a lack of funds.

(6) "SPEND DOWN your assets and apply for MEDICAID, as that system is being used and in place and easier to administer.

INTERMEDIATE CARE

A plea for VA to contract with Maui Adult Day Care Center. John has found an incentive to do more than stay in his recliner despairing over his loss of vision. He attends MADCC 5 days a week where he has found new friends, activities, exercise and new interests. It is a safe environment where his self-worth has been restored as he helps others. "Health" is more than physical rehabilitation, the mental, emotional social and psychological aspect is so important and present at MADCC. John has found a second home. MADCC have centers in Kahului, Lahaina, and Hana . Add "Health" to their name.

In conclusion:

Maui County's service members serving in Iraq and elsewhere are contacted and made aware of their Veteran Rights. Included is the Dept. of the Army's (DS3) disabled Soldiers Support System for the severely disabled. Soldiers include Reservists and National Guard and their families. Support is offered throughout notification, treatment and eventual return to home station and home destination. It is the home destination segment we should be concerned with. How and where will these veterans fit into the health care systems of the outer islands?

Where will the funds come from to support on or islands, the VA Health Care that is available only on Oahu? You should not provide for the outer islands at the expense of care on Oahu, but you must find ways to provide better VA Health Care in Maui County. WE PLEAD FOR COMPASSIONATE SOLUTIONS!

Mahalo for listening and for your caring.

PREPARED STATEMENT OF DON DICKENSHEET

Howzit from the island of Lanai and yesterday I got a copy of a letter from Mr. Obado about a hearing well please allow me to throw my 2 cents in if I may as my name is Don Dickensheet and I have lived on Lanai since retiring from the Navy after 21 years in 1992 and let me first tell you that the only thing you can do successfully on Lanai when it comes to medical is die! Almost everything else you have to go to Honolulu for, don't get me wrong those of us who live here realize this and the pleasure we gain from living on this island outweighs a lot of the alternatives.

In August of 2000 I like Mr. Obado suffered a cerebral aneurysm and have since then been stumbling along and in this day of the internet I don't feel I should have to sell my home here and move to some squalid apartment in San Diego to get my benefits, as we here on Lanai realize we are ALWAYS on the low end of the pecking order as they have vans in Honolulu to whisk all the guys living in the bushes on Nimitz highway up to the Sparky VA center to dry out for a few weeks most folks here just give up after awhile and I can understand their frustration getting up at 0 dark thirty to dial 1–800 numbers and talk to machine during normal working hours in DC. After my aneurysm I started thinking now that my life was ruined.

Why had this happened and it took me 3 years to prove to the VA that it was service connected because unknown to me the whole time I was on active duty I was growing a brain tumor which they failed to detect as it caused a hearing loss in my left ear and they never bothered to fully investigate the cause on my retirement physical so with only Bill Station to help me once a month I got busy and it took 3 years but I got it done and am now in the process of trying to get a grant to have a new bathroom made as when I first came home from the hospital I spent out of my own pocket for grab bars a new toilet etc. only to find out later on that the VA will provide it. To this date, we are still working on this and all I ever seem to get is forms requesting more forms? My rating decision has already been made and I don't know what the hang up is but since I refuse to play the Press 1 for English and press 2 to listen to goofy music game I guess it will take me another 3 years at least to get what I am entitled to. My heart goes out to the old timers here whose families would have to play these games when they pass away to get them buried here in our veterans cemetery.

We NEED a central place here on Lanai where vets can go and actually speak to a human being who knows how to get their benefits. For example, I would like to see someone get hold of NALCO in Honolulu and see if regular logistic flights could be scheduled to all islands utilizing the C–12 aircraft which Navy pilots utilize while on shore duty to maintain flight quals and instead of flying in circles around the runway doing touch and goes how about flying to Molokai, Lanai Maui and the Big Island to pick up vets for their appointments in Honolulu saving the $200 plus. There are many ways that already exist within the system to accommodate us and in my case being retired military it really burnt me up to HAVE to spend $400 to go re-new my wife's ID card in Honolulu bet Dan doesn't do this? Also let me get back to the retired thing we military retirees give up a lot to live on outer islands as we don't get to buy cheap gas, food, and clothing and we all know this when we make the decision to live where we do but it really smarts when we cant even get the basic entitlements which we were promised and there are probably less than a dozen military retirees on this island but each one of us has to do something different to try to get our benefits as we know so much more how the system works than those vets who only were in for one hitch, they earned these benefits many paid with their own blood and to act as if they don't exist because they chose to live in a place that doesn't fit in the required block, example one form I use to get repaid my co-payments for Medication has DO NOT USE PO BOX on it for address guess the bean counters don't know that zip code 96763 is PO BOX ONLY I think I got that through their heads by telling them to dial 1–800– ASK–USPS its stupid stuff like this that cause delays for months! I for one would like to get all Vets on the same page here so we can get what we earned.

Prepared Statement of Francine Atwell

I am the wife of a disabled vet and I have recently become disabled myself, due in part to my husband's severing PTSD.

The VA provides very little support to veterans' families. On Maui, there is a women's/spouse group primarily focused on understanding our veterans PTSD but it is not enough, even though the meeting has been a very good start.

First families pay the high-test emotional price sometimes even higher than veterans themselves for the veteran's injuries and illness. We need more help to withstand the stress that comes with long-term conditions.

Second, the families are true first responders to our veterans.

Given the opportunities to lean assertive training/communications skills or anger management techniques not for ourselves and for our vets. We can deal with our vets more effectively and as caregivers reinforce VA care.

Supporting the families supports the vet in very cost effective way. Group meeting and classes are very expensive compared to the costs of hospital treatment and the effects of abuse and violence which is very real to many of us.

Prepared Statement of Sgt. Albert A. Newsham

I want to know why the thousands of combat veterans are not permitted to collect "combat related special compensation." I was forced to retired from the Army because of my wounds. I spent my time in combat. I spent 2 and half years in Army hospitals and I am 100 percent disabled.

Let's be fair, we did what you asked us to do. We went when you said Vietnam and our country needed us. Now it is time for you to step up and do the correct and honorable thing. Show us you can keep your word. Pass the legislation so men and women like me can receive the compensation we earned with our blood and tears and honor.

A P E N D I X 2

PREPARED STATEMENT OF JONATHAN A. PERLIN, MD, PHD, MSHA, FACP, UNDER SECRETARY FOR HEALTH DEPARTMENT OF VETERANS AFFAIRS

Mr. Chairman and Members of the Committee, mahalo nui loa for the opportunity to appear before you today to discuss the state of VA care in Hawaii. It is a privilege to be here on Kauai—the Garden Isle—to speak and answer questions about issues important to veterans residing in Hawaii.

First, Mr. Chairman, I would like to thank you for your outstanding leadership and advocacy on behalf of our Nation's veterans. During your tenure as Chairman of this Committee, you have clearly demonstrated your commitment to veterans by acting decisively to ensure the needs of veterans are met. In addition, I appreciate your interest in and support of the Department of Veterans Affairs (VA).

I also would like to express my appreciation and respect for Senator Akaka, Ranking Member of this Committee. Along with his colleague, Senator Inouye, Senator Akaka has done so much for the veterans residing in Hawaii and other islands in the Pacific region. As I will highlight later, his vision, guidance and assistance have directly led to an unprecedented level of health care services for veterans, construction of state-of-the-art facilities in Honolulu and remarkable improvements in access to health care services for veterans residing on neighbor islands, including Kauai.

Today, I will briefly review the VA Sierra Pacific Network that includes Hawaii and the Pacific region; provide an overview of the VA Pacific Islands Health Care System (VAPIHCS) and the VA clinic here in Kauai; highlight issues of particular interest to veterans residing in Kauai, including the availability of long-term care services, specialty care and access to the VA clinic from the west side of Kauai; and address any questions posed by Members of the Committee.

VA SIERRA PACIFIC NETWORK (VISN 21)

The VA Sierra Pacific Network (Veterans Integrated Service Network [VISN] 21) is one of 21 integrated health care networks in the Veterans Health Administration (VHA). The VA Sierra Pacific Network provides services to veterans residing in Hawaii and the Pacific Basin (including the Philippines, Guam, American Samoa and Commonwealth of the Northern Marianas Islands), northern Nevada and central/ northern California. There are an estimated 1.25 million veterans living within the boundaries of the VA Sierra Pacific Network.

The VA Sierra Pacific Network includes six major health care systems based in Honolulu, HI; Palo Alto, CA; San Francisco, CA; Sacramento, CA; Fresno, CA and Reno, NV. Dr. Robert Wiebe serves as director and oversees clinical and administrative operations throughout the Network. In Fiscal Year 2005 (FY05), the Network provided services to 227,000 veterans. There were about 2.8 million clinic stops and 24,000 inpatient admissions. The cumulative full-time employment equivalents (FTEE) level was 8,200 and the operating budget was about $1.3 billion, which is an increase of $378 million since 2001.

The VA Sierra Pacific Network is remarkable in several ways. In fiscal year 2005, the Network was the only VISN in VHA to meet the performance targets for all six Clinical Interventions that directly address adherence to evidence-based clinical practice. The Network hosts 11 (out of 65) VHA Centers of Excellence-the most in VHA. The VA Sierra Pacific Network also has the highest funded research programs in VHA. Finally, VISN 21 operates one of four Polytrauma units that are dedicated to addressing the clinical needs of the most severely wounded Operation Iraqi Freedom/Operation Enduring Freedom (OIF/OEF) veterans.

VA PACIFIC ISLANDS HEALTH CARE SYSTEM (VAPIHCS)

As noted above, VAPIHCS is one of six major health care systems in VISN 21. VAPIHCS is unique in several important aspects: its vast catchment area covering 2.6 million square-miles (including Hawaii, Guam, American Samoa and Commonwealth of the Northern Marianas); island topography and the challenges to access it creates; richness of the culture of Pacific Islanders; and the ethnic diversity of patients and staff. In fiscal year 2005, there were an estimated 113,000 veterans living in Hawaii (9 percent of Network total).

VAPIHCS provides care in six locations: Ambulatory Care Center (ACC) and Center for Aging (CFA) on the campus of the Tripler Army Medical Center (AMC) in Honolulu; and community-based outpatient clinics (CBOCs) in Lihue (Kauai), Kahului (Maui), Kailua-Kona (Hawaii), Hilo (Hawaii) and Agana (Guam). VAPIHCS also sends clinicians and support staff from these locations to provide services on Lanai, Molokai and American Samoa. The inpatient post-traumatic stress disorder (PTSD) unit formerly in Hilo is in the process of relocating to Honolulu. In addition to VAPIHCS, VHA operates five Readjustment Counseling Centers (Vet Centers) in Honolulu, Lihue, Wailuku, Kailua-Kona and Hilo that provide counseling, psychosocial support and outreach.

Dr. James Hastings was recently appointed Director, VAPIHCS. Dr. Hastings has impressive credentials, including tenure as Chair, Department of Medicine, John A. Burns School of Medicine, University of Hawaii, and Commanding General at Walter Reed AMC and Tripler AMC. I am excited about the possibilities that his tenure as Director at VAPIHCS brings.

In fiscal year 2005, VAPIHCS provided services to 18,300 veterans in Hawaii (8 percent of Network total). There were 194,000 clinic stops in Hawaii during fiscal year 2005 (7 percent of Network total), an increase of 36 percent since fiscal year 00. The cumulative FTEE for the health care system was 478 employees. The budget for VAPIHCS (including General Purpose, Specific Purpose and Medical Care Cost Funds [MCCF]) has increased from $53 million in fiscal year 1999 to $102 million in fiscal year 2005 (about 8 percent of Network total). In addition, VISN 21 provided over $20 million in supplemental funds to VAPIHCS over the past two Fiscal Years to ensure VAPIHCS met its financial obligations.

VAPIHCS provides or contracts for a comprehensive array of health care services. VAPIHCS directly provides primary care, including preventive services and health screenings, and mental health services at all locations. Selected specialty services are also currently provided at the Honolulu campus and to a lesser extent, at CBOCs. VAPIHCS recently hired specialists in gero-psychiatry, gastroenterology, ophthalmology and radiology. VAPIHCS is actively recruiting additional specialists in cardiology, orthopedic surgery and urology. Inpatient long-term care is available at the 60–bed Center for Aging. Inpatient mental health services are provided by VA staff on a 20-bed ward within Tripler AMC and at the 16-bed PTSD Residential Rehabilitation Program (PRRP) that was formerly in Hilo (now relocating to Honolulu). VAPIHCS contracts for care with DoD (at Tripler AMC and Guam Naval Hospital) and community facilities for inpatient medical-surgical care.

The current constellation of VA facilities and services represents a remarkable transformation over the past several years. Previously, the VAPIHCS (formerly known as the VA Medical and Regional Office Center [VAMROC] Honolulu) operated primary care and mental health clinics based in the Prince Kuhio Federal Building in downtown Honolulu and CBOCs on the neighbor islands that were staffed primarily with nurse practitioners. Senator Akaka and his colleagues in Congress approved $83 million in Major Construction funds to build a state-of-the-art ambulatory care center and nursing home care unit on the Tripler AMC campus and these facilities were activated in 2000 and 1997, respectively. VISN 21 allocated nearly $17 million from FY98–FY00 to activate these projects. VISN 21 also provided dedicated funds (e.g., $2 million in fiscal year 2001) to enhance care on the neighbor islands by expanding/renovating clinic space and adding additional staff to ensure there are primary care physicians and psychiatrists at all CBOCs.

KAUAI CBOC

VA operates a community-based outpatient clinic (CBOC), located in Lihue (3–3367 Kuhio Highway, Suite 200, Lihue, HI, 96766–1061). In fiscal year 2003, VAPIHCS spent $470,000 to renovate the clinic. The Kauai Vet Center is co-located with the clinic in Lihue.

CBOCs, like the one here in Kauai, play a crucial role in the care of veterans in Hawaii. Since they are located in small communities, CBOCs have the feel of an old-fashioned doctor's office. Patients get to know their caregivers (in ways not possible in a large medical center) and clinic staff gets to know their patients, including their friends, military stories and even their grandchildren's names. Staff at the Kauai CBOC sees its role as not just caregiver, but also as an active participant in the local community. On its own time, staff participates in community events like Veterans Day, Fourth of July celebrations and December holiday festivities.

The Kauai CBOC serves an estimated island veteran population in fiscal year 2005 of 5,420. In fiscal year 2005, 1,518 veterans were enrolled for care and 1,016 veterans received care ("users") at the Kauai CBOC. The market penetrations for enrollees and "users" are 28 percent and 18 percent, respectively, and compare favorably with rates within VISN 21 and VHA.

The current authorized full-time employment equivalents (FTEE) level is 9.0, including a full-time primary care physician, psychiatrist and nurse practitioner, and all positions are filled. With this staff, the Kauai CBOC provides a broad range of primary care and mental health services. In addition, VAPIHCS provides specialty care services at the clinic by sending VA staff from Honolulu and other VA facilities in California. Services provided by clinicians traveling to Kauai include cardiology, nephrology, neurology, optometry, orthopedics, rheumatology and urology. If veterans need services not available at the clinic, VAPIHCS arranges and pays for care in the local community (e.g., Wilcox Hospital), Honolulu (including Tripler AMC) or VA facilities in California. In fiscal year 2005, VA spent more than $2.1 million for non-VA care in the private sector (i.e., not including costs at other VA or DoD facilities) for residents of Kauai.

In fiscal year 2005, the Kauai CBOC recorded 6,024 clinic stops, representing a 35 percent increase from fiscal year 2000 (i.e., 4,457 stops). The clinic has short waiting times for new patients with very few veterans waiting more than 30 days for their first primary care appointment.

SPECIAL ISSUES

Long-term care. As a group, the veteran population is aging. Consequently, long-term care (LTC) services are a very important component of the continuum of care provided by VA. VA provides both inpatient LTC (i.e., institutional care) and non-institutional care (NIC). VA's approach to LTC is to provide extended care services in the least restrictive setting that is appropriate for the clinical condition of the veteran and his/her personal circumstances.

As an alternative to inpatient LTC, VA has developed and fostered a variety of NIC programs. NIC includes Adult Day Health Care (ADHC), Contract Adult Day Health Care (CADHC), Home-based Primary Care (HBPC), Contract Home Health Care (CHHC), Homemaker/Home Health Aid (H/HHA), Home Hospice, Home Respite, Geriatric Evaluation and Management (GEM) Program and Spinal Cord Injury (SCI) Home Program. Secretary Nicholson and his predecessors authorized the expansion of VA's NIC services. The capacity of these programs has grown rapidly since fiscal year 1998 and VA is expecting a further increase of 18 percent in fiscal year 2006.

This trend is also present in Hawaii. In fiscal year 2005, VAPIHCS recorded a NIC ADC of 108 patients, representing an increase of 38 percent compared to fiscal year 2004 (i.e., NIC ADC 78.2 patients). In some locations in Hawaii, VA directly provides NIC services. In other venues, including Kauai, VA contracts for these services. The following table displays trend in VAPIHCS obligations for LTC services in the community.

Trend in Non-VA Expenditures at VAPIHCS
[$000]

FY 2002	FY 2003	FY 2004	FY 2005	Change FY 2002–FY 2005
Comunity nursing home (CNH)				
$93	$280	$661	$1,047	442%
Non-institutional care (NIC)				
$97	$126	$191	$716	638%

The decision to "make or buy" is based on the clinical need for and availability of these services in the local community. These decisions are re-evaluated based on changes in workload and availability of resources. As an example, VAPIHCS currently operates HBPC programs in the Big Island (i.e., at its CBOCs in Hilo and

Kailua-Kona, but not in Kauai or Maui. VAPIHCS is currently reassessing the feasibility of adding staff at its CBOCs here in Kauai and Maui to provide HBPC.

At the request of Senator Akaka, the Office of Inspector General recently began a review of access to NIC in VHA. Although its findings and recommendations are not yet available, I am already taking actions in Hawaii to ensure clinical and eligibility criteria are correctly applied. As an example, VAPIHCS had been inappropriately restricting H/HHA services to veterans meeting the eligibility requirements for mandatory inpatient LTC as set forth in the Veterans Millennium Health Care and Benefits Act (Millennium Act), Public Law 106–117 (1999). These local eligibility restrictions have been rescinded.

Nursing home care is reserved for situations in which the veteran can no longer safely be cared for at home. VA is committed to providing nursing home care to all veterans for whom such care is mandated by the Millennium Act (i.e., 70 percent or more service-connected rating or requiring nursing home care because of a service-connected disability). VA will continue to provide long-term maintenance care to other veterans on a discretionary basis as resources permit. VA provides inpatient LTC services directly in its nursing home care facilities, pays for nursing home care in communities and supports State Veterans Homes (with construction funds and per diem reimbursements).

As noted earlier, VAPIHCS operates a long-term care inpatient unit in Honolulu. Recently, this 60-bed unit operates close to its capacity (e.g., in fiscal year 2005, the average daily census [ADC] was 56 patients). VA has contracts with and places veterans in two community nursing home care units in Oahu. In fiscal year 2005, VAPIHCS spent more than $1 million in community nursing home (CNH) care-nearly quadruple the amount spent in fiscal year 2003 (i.e., $280 thousand). VAPIHCS is interested in expanding its CNH program, but unfortunately, the other community facilities (including those on Neighbor Islands) VAPIHCS has contacted do not meet VA's life and safety codes or are unwilling to fulfill the requirements of VA's CNH contract.

VA is also providing funding and working with the State of Hawaii to build and activate the first State Veterans Home in Hawaii. The 95-bed nursing home facility will be built in Hilo at the site of the former Hilo Hospital on the Hilo Medical Center Campus. The cost estimate for the project is $31 million and VA is contributing 65 percent (i.e., $20 million).

Specialty services. The size of the veteran population and number of VA patients limit the feasibility of having a large cadre of medical and surgical specialists based in the Kauai CBOC. Nonetheless, VA recognizes that some veterans in Kauai have needs that go beyond primary care and mental health. As I noted earlier, VA sends specialists from Honolulu and California to the clinic on a regular basis. Services provided by clinicians traveling to Kauai include cardiology, nephrology, neurology, optometry, orthopedics, rheumatology and urology. VAPIHCS also refers patients to the local community for care at VA expense (when eligibility criteria are met) and transports (also at VA expense when eligibility criteria are met) patients to the VA facility in Honolulu.

VAPIHCS is utilizing telehealth technology to expand access to specialty care (e.g., dermatology). VAPIHCS estimates that telehealth services are provided more than 10 hours per week at the Kauai CBOC. As additional specialists are hired at the VA facility based in Honolulu, these clinicians will be able to travel to Kauai and further utilize telehealth technologies.

West Kauai. Although Kauai is a relatively small island (i.e., 550 square-miles), transportation on the island can be problematic. As an example, the driving time from the west side of Kauai to the VA clinic can be up to an hour. VAPIHCS estimates approximately 190 existing patients (i.e., "current users") live on the west side of Kauai. Consequently, it is not practical to establish a new clinic on the west side or rotate staff from the existing clinic. Instead, VA will work with community organizations, such as veterans' service organizations, and local government to enhance transportation options for veterans.

CONCLUSION

In summary, with the support of Senator Akaka and other Members of Congress, VA is providing an unprecedented level of health care services to veterans residing in Hawaii and the Pacific Region. VA now has state-of-the-art facilities and enhanced services in Honolulu, as well as robust staffing on the neighbor islands and has expanded or renovated clinics in many locations. VA is bringing more specialists on board and preparing for the newest generation of veterans-those who bravely served in southwest Asia.

VAPIHCS still faces several challenges, in part due to the topography of its catchment area. VAPIHCS will meet these challenges by utilizing telehealth technologies, sharing specialists, developing new delivery models and opening new clinics as demographics suggest and resources allow. I am proud of the improvements in VA services in Hawaii, but recognize that our job is not done.

Again, Mr. Chairman and other members of the Committee, mahalo nui loa for the opportunity to testify at this hearing. I would be delighted to address any questions you may have for me or other members of the panel.

PREPARED STATEMENT OF ROBERT SHAW, NATIONAL LEGISLATIVE CHAIRMAN
NATIONAL ASSOCIATION OF STATE VETERANS HOMES

Chairman Craig, Senator Akaka and other Distinguished Members:

Thank you for the opportunity given to me to present the views of the National Association of State Veterans Homes before this hearing of the Committee on Veterans' Affairs. It is an honor to join you today on this beautiful island of Kauai to explore ideas and seek methods to better serve Hawaii's aging veterans with long-term care services they need and have earned through their service.

I am presenting testimony today on behalf of the National Association of State Veterans Homes (NASVH), an all-volunteer, non-profit organization founded over a half century ago to promote the common interests of State veterans homes and the deserving elderly veterans and their families that we serve. The membership of NASVH consists of the administrators and senior staffs of State-operated veterans homes throughout the United States. Our current membership includes 119 homes in 47 States and the Commonwealth of Puerto Rico. We provide nursing home care in 114 homes, domiciliary care in 52 of those locations, and hospital-type care in five of our homes. Our State homes presently provide over 27,500 resident beds for veterans, of which more than 21,000 are nursing home beds. I am here today as both the National Legislative Chairman of NASVH, an elected position I have held since the year 2000, and also as the Administrator of the State Veterans Center in Rifle, Colorado, where we provide skilled nursing care to 100 veterans and family members each day.

The State home program dates back to the post-Civil War era when several States established homes in which to provide domicile, shelter and care to homeless, sick and maimed Union soldiers and sailors. In 1888 Congress first authorized Federal grants-in-aid to States that maintained these homes, including a per diem allowance for each veteran of twenty-seven cents ($100 per year per veteran). Over the years since that time, the State home program has been expanded and refined to reflect the improvements in standards of medical practice, including the advent of nursing home, domiciliary, adult day health, and other specialized geriatric care for veterans. For example, the facility that I manage in Colorado now includes a Special Care Unit for Alzheimer's and dementia patients, a growing need in this population. There are also now two State homes providing adult day health care, and a number of others are developing programs in this new discipline and other emerging approaches to delivering care in less restrictive settings.

Today, the State home program is supported in two ways by the Federal Government: through per diem subsidy payments that help States cover daily costs, and construction grants to keep our homes up-to-date and safe for our patients and staffs. Subject to appropriations, VA provides construction matching-grant funding for up to 65 percent of the cost of constructing or rehabilitating homes, with at least 35 percent covered by State funding commitments. The per diem program provides reimbursement to State homes, currently $63.40 for nursing home care, which is about 30 percent of the average cost to the States. Section 1741 of Title 38, United States Code, authorizes VA to provide a per diem rate of up to 50 percent of the States' average daily cost, but VA has not been able to bring the actual rate paid to our homes near this statutory cost ceiling.

Mr. Chairman, as you well know, the last budget debate for fiscal year 2006 was a crucial one for the State home program. We want to thank this Committee, and especially you, Mr. Chairman and Senator Akaka, for the vital role you both played in defending the State home program during the budget and appropriations cycle just concluded for fiscal year 2006. Thanks to your leadership, as well as tremendous support and leadership from Senators Hutchison, Feinstein and others, the Administration's proposals to dramatically restrict per diem payments to only a small portion of the veterans currently in our homes, and to impose a moratorium on further construction funding, were soundly rejected. We are grateful that Congress spoke clearly and forcefully on theses matters in the Joint Explanatory Statement accompanying the Act:

The conferees do not agree with the proposal contained in the budget to alter the long-term care policies, including a policy of priority care in nursing homes. The conferees have provided with this total appropriation, sufficient resources to maintain a policy of providing long-term care to all veterans, utilizing VA-owned facilities, community nursing homes, State nursing homes, and other non-institutional venues. The conferees expect there to be no change from the policies in existence prior to fiscal year 2005.

We look forward to working closely with you in this New Year should we again face budgetary and legislative challenges during the Second Session of the 109th Congress.

Today, however, we are focusing on how best to provide long term care services to Hawaii's veterans who need and deserve this care. As I stated previously, 47 States already have at least one state veterans home in operation, leaving just three states—Hawaii, Alaska and Delaware—which do not. Of course, as you well know, there is a new 95-bed State veterans' home under construction in Hilo on the Big Island scheduled to open later this year that will substantially meet the needs of veterans residing on that island. In addition, long-term care and transitional rehabilitative services are being provided now on Oahu by a VA-operated, 60-bed Center for Aging, located at Tripler Army Medical Center. The VA Center for Aging will partially meet Honolulu-area veterans' long term care needs, but additional resources will probably be needed on that island as the elderly Oahu veteran population continues to grow.

There remain, however, significant gaps in long term care services to Hawaii's veterans due to the nature and geography of this great State. In particular, the Neighbor Islands, with their smaller overall veteran populations and physical separation, face a much more difficult challenge in trying to meet the needs of their frail, elderly veterans. For those living on Kauai, Molokai, Maui and other Neighbor Islands, the facilities at Hilo and Oahu simply are not realistic options. The question before this panel today is how best to meet these needs given the challenges we have identified and the inevitable budgetary constraints faced by VA and Congress.

Under current law, as set forth in Public Law 106–117, the Veterans Millennium Health Care and Benefits Act, Congress established specific criteria for authorizing construction of new State homes. It is possible under VA criteria that Hawaii, in addition to building the new home at Hilo, could justify building another State home with about 120 beds based upon its State-wide veteran population. However, given the unique island geography of Hawaii, with vast seas separating islands, as well as their rich cultural traditions, it would not be practical to expect veterans from close-knit families and communities on one island to leave their families and travel great distances to another island for long-term care. While the construction of a second State veterans' home somewhere in Hawaii might solve one island's problem for aging veterans, it would not adequately address their lack of long-term care services on other islands.

For better or for worse, Mr. Chairman, Hawaii is not alone in trying to address the challenge of meeting the needs of geographically dispersed populations. Other large rural States, including, Alaska, Wyoming, Montana and Idaho, among others, face similar problems in trying to provide high quality and convenient long term care for veterans who live at great distances from larger population centers and major VA facilities. As Congress and VA seek to address this problem, it could prove beneficial for this Committee to look at how Alaska, our largest State, has managed this challenge.

Over the years, Alaska's State government, Congress and Alaska's veterans' organizations have considered numerous proposals for that State to seek VA matching grants for the construction of State homes for veterans, but no concrete proposal was ever approved by the Governor or the State legislature. This is not to suggest that Alaska has no facilities serving older veterans in need of long-term care.

Beginning in 1913 in the city of Sitka, the State of Alaska began operating what are called "Pioneer Homes." Today, Alaska operates six of these homes providing more than 500 total long term care beds in Sitka, Anchorage, Fairbanks, Juneau, Ketchikan and Palmer. These homes provide nursing and residential care to "Alaska Pioneers" — any Alaska citizen over age 65, in declining health, and in need of significant care for activities of daily living. These homes are supported by State funds, insurance reimbursements and private payments, very similar to the mixed financing arrangements of State veterans' homes. Although these homes are not solely reserved for veterans, about one-quarter of the residents are veterans of military service.

In the past decade, Alaska's "Pioneer Homes" also have become licensed assisted living facilities, offering a comprehensive range of services to meet the needs of the elderly residents. Professional services cover the full range of needed care, including assistance with activities of daily living, skilled nursing, and compassionate end-of-life services. Many Pioneer residents receive a level of service that would otherwise be delivered in a hospital, a traditional nursing home, a hospice, or in a home-based elder program under a Medicaid waiver arrangement Alaska reached with the Center for Medicare and Medicaid Services (CMS).

In May 2004, Congress passed legislation to define the Alaska "Pioneer Homes" as a single State veterans home for purposes of establishing eligibility for participation in VA's State home programs. Based upon this legislation, Alaska submitted a request for, and was approved for, the construction of a 79-bed veterans' domiciliary as a new wing to the existing Pioneer Home in Palmer, Alaska. Construction of this new wing began this past summer and is expected to be completed late this year.

Similar to Alaska, Hawaii's dispersed veteran population on the smaller islands generally cannot justify construction of veterans' homes on each island. However, using the Alaska Pioneer Home concept as a foundation, it may be feasible to advance legislation deeming a similar status to the Hawaii Health Systems Corporation (HHSC)—as one "State veterans' home" for purposes of HHSC's participation in the VA State veterans' home programs. The HHSC, a public benefit corporation, is an extensive hospital system of 12 facilities on five islands, and is the largest health provider in the Neighbor Islands. Under this scenario, smaller bed units—perhaps ten to thirty beds each, depending on local circumstances—could be justified under existing VA criteria in a manner similar to the Alaska model. Such projects could be developed as separate facilities within these existing State-owned and operated hospitals to accommodate the needs of elder and disabled Hawaii veterans in rural and remote locations.

Mr. Chairman, like you, NASVH is committed to meeting the long-term care needs of veterans, whether they live in major metropolitan areas or in geographically dispersed areas such as these Neighbor Islands of Hawaii. Although Hawaii may not be able to cost-effectively justify the establishment of large, stand-alone State veterans' nursing homes on each of the Neighbor Islands, other creative solutions such as the Pioneer Homes model may be worth pursuing. NASVH stands ready to work with you, this Committee, Congress and VA to meet the diverse needs of veterans living throughout Hawaii, as well as other veterans living in large States such as Alaska, Wyoming, Montana, and Idaho.

Mr. Chairman, Senator Akaka, and other Members the Committee, once again I want to thank you for allowing me to testify here today on behalf of the National Association of State Veterans Homes. We look forward to working with you and the Congress to strengthen, rather than weaken, this foundation of veterans' long-term care. The care provided by our member homes is an indispensable, cost-effective, and successful element in VA's provision of comprehensive health care. We are grateful for your past support and hope that should we see a repetition of the misguided budget proposals submitted by the Administration last year, that we can again count on your support. Millions of veterans are going to need long-term care in the years ahead. We want to be sure that the State home program is there to support them.

Mr. Chairman, this concludes my testimony. I would be pleased to answer any questions you may have on this or other topics in which I might be helpful to the Committee.

PREPARED STATEMENT OF EDWARD KAWAMURA, VETERAN

To: Senator Craig, Ranking Member, Senator Akaka, and Members of this hearing.

My name is Edward M. Kawamura. I am a Vietnam Veteran who retired from the U.S. Army in 1978. I have been involved with veterans and families as Department of Hawaii, Disabled American Veteran Commander, Kauai Veteran's Council President, Board Member Office of Veterans Services, and current Board member to the VA Advisory Board.

The services that are provided by our VA are "No. 1." The personnel at the Kauai Community Based Outpatient Clinic (CBOC) are the best. Their professionalism, dedication, and willingness to help, make them the best. Their rating by JACCO reflects their No. 1 rating. I applaud all the workers involved at the CBOC and VET Center.

There are some improvements and visions that I would like to share as improvements and new programs for Kauai Veterans. They are as follows:

a. *Manpower.* More manpower is needed. A Home Healthcare Nurse is needed. Our aging population, coupled with problems of getting veterans to the medical clinic, mandates the need to provide the care and services at the homes. This nurse would help in reducing time now serviced by our doctor and nurse practitioner so more veterans can be served and reduce scheduling time for appointments. Outreach programs are needed, and can be accomplished with more manpower. Increased manpower and services are needed also due to the increased veteran population returning from the Iraqi War.

b. *Facility.* The CBOC has outgrown itself. The size and space for the waiting room, screening rooms, prescription vault and conference rooms needs to be increased. Parking is another area that needs to be increased. Recommendation: A new CBOC be constructed at the Kauai Veterans Center site. Parking is adequate and space is available for new building. This would make for a "One-Stop" veterans operation.

c. *Funding.* More funds should be made available for travel as our VA has a huge geographic area to cover. All of these travels must be by air. Care servers, care givers, and patients are often required to travel to provide or receive services.

d. *Kauai Veterans Cemetery.* Phase I expansion by the VA doubled the size of the cemetery. They did not provide for increase in manpower or equipment. This should be a factor included in future plans.

e. *Vision.* The vision is that there should be an Old Soldiers Home of the Pacific here on Kauai. The aged veterans who have nowhere to go should be afforded a place to live out their lives. This is so we can accommodate the Pacific Rim veterans to provide for an environment similar to their lifestyles. The site location at Sam Mahelona Hospital has the ideal view and environmental elements for a good soldier's home.

The Spark M. Matsunaga Medical Center is a perfect example that reflects the dedication by our congressional and your committee to our fellow veterans. This facility is "No. 1."

I would like to thank each and everyone on your committee for taking time to hear our concerns. This is truly the only way to hear first hand the needs of our fellow veterans and their families. Thank you very much.

United States Government Accountability Office

GAO

Testimony

Before the Committee on Veterans'
Affairs, U.S. Senate

For Release on Delivery
Expected at 10:00 a.m. HST
Lihue, Hawaii
Monday, January 9, 2006

VA LONG-TERM CARE

Trends and Planning Challenges in Providing Nursing Home Care to Veterans

Statement of Laurie E. Ekstrand
Director, Health Care

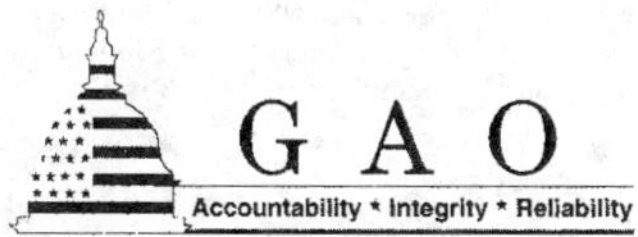

GAO-06-333T

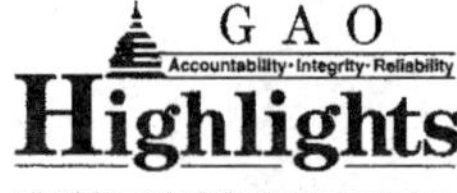

Highlights

Highlights of GAO-06-333T, a testimony before the Committee on Veterans' Affairs, U.S. Senate

VA LONG-TERM CARE

Trends and Planning Challenges in Providing Nursing Home Care to Veterans

Why GAO Did This Study

The Department of Veterans Affairs (VA) operates a nursing home program that provides or pays for veterans' care in three nursing home settings: VA-operated nursing homes, community nursing homes, and state veterans' nursing homes. In addition, veterans needing nursing home care may also receive it from non-VA providers that are not funded by VA. VA is faced with a large elderly veteran population, many of whom may be in need of nursing home care. In 2004, 38 percent of the nation's veteran population was over the age of 65, compared with 12 percent of the general population. The Veterans Millennium Health Care and Benefits Act (Millennium Act) of 1999 and VA policy require that VA provide nursing home care to certain veterans.

This statement focuses on VA's nursing home program and trends in nursing home expenditures, trends in the number of patients served, or "patient workload," and key challenges VA faces in planning for nursing home care for veterans.

To examine these trends, GAO updated information from prior work with spending and patient workload data for fiscal year 2005 that VA provided. In a November 2004 report, GAO presented spending and patient workload data through fiscal year 2003. GAO discussed the updated information with VA and incorporated comments as appropriate.

www.gao.gov/cgi-bin/getrpt?GAO-06-333T.

To view the full product, including the scope and methodology, click on the link above. For more information, contact Laurie E. Ekstrand at (202) 512-7101 or ekstrandl@gao.gov.

What GAO Found

VA's reported overall nursing home care expenditures in its three settings increased from $2.3 billion to almost $3.2 billion from fiscal year 2003 through fiscal year 2005. VA officials attributed the expenditure increase from fiscal year 2003 to fiscal year 2005, in part, to a change in the cost accounting system used to develop expenditure totals for each nursing home setting. Based on VA's reported expenditures, VA-operated nursing homes continued to account for about three-quarters of VA's overall nursing home care expenditures in fiscal year 2005, as they did in fiscal year 2003. In fiscal year 2005, 77 percent of nursing home care expenditures were accounted for by VA-operated nursing homes, compared to 73 percent in 2003. VA spent the remainder on state veterans' nursing homes and community nursing homes. From fiscal year 2003 through fiscal year 2005, the percentage of overall expenditures for state veterans' nursing homes declined from 15 to 12 percent and the percentage of overall expenditures for community nursing homes declined from 12 to 11 percent.

VA's overall patient workload in nursing homes increased to an average of 34,375 patients per day by fiscal year 2005, 3.5 percent above the fiscal year 2003 workload. State veterans' nursing homes accounted for over half of VA's patient workload in fiscal year 2005. The workload percent is higher than the 12 percent expenditure in state veterans' nursing homes partly because VA pays on average about one-third of the costs for care veterans receive in state veterans' nursing homes, compared to the full cost in other settings. From fiscal year 2003 through fiscal year 2005, the percentage of workload provided in state veterans' nursing homes increased from 50 to 52 percent. In contrast, the percentage of patient workload provided in VA-operated nursing homes declined from 37 to 35 percent. The percentage of workload in community nursing homes stayed the same at 13 percent.

VA faces two key challenges in planning for the provision of nursing home care. The first challenge is estimating who will seek care from VA and what their nursing home care needs will be. This includes estimating the number of veterans that will be eligible for nursing home care, based on law and VA policy, and the extent to which these veterans will be seeking care for short-stay postacute needs or long-stay chronic needs. A second key challenge VA faces is determining whether it will maintain or increase the proportion of nursing home care demand it meets in each of the three nursing home settings or whether veterans will need to rely more on other non-VA nursing home care providers that are funded by other programs, such as Medicaid and Medicare.

Mr. Chairman and Members of the Committee:

We are pleased to be here today as you discuss issues regarding the Department of Veterans Affairs (VA) health care program for veterans. One important part of that program is nursing home care, which accounts for about 9 percent of VA's health care expenditures. The VA nursing home program provides care in three settings. It operates its own nursing homes in 134 locations, including a nursing home in Honolulu; it pays for care under contract in non-VA nursing homes, referred to as community nursing homes, including two community nursing homes on the island of Oahu; and it pays about one-third of the costs per day for veterans in state veterans' nursing homes, one of which will be built in Hilo.[1] In addition, veterans needing nursing home care may also receive it from non-VA providers that are not funded by VA. In its three settings, a range of nursing home services is provided to veterans, including short-stay postacute care for patients recovering from a condition such as a stroke to long-stay care for patients who cannot be cared for at home because of severe, chronic physical or mental limitations. VA nursing home care is part of a continuum of long-term care services that VA provides, including services to veterans in the community and in veterans' own homes.[2]

As you know, meeting veterans' nursing home care needs is a key issue for VA nationally, and here in Hawaii, because of the large elderly veteran population, many of whom are in need of such care. Nationwide, the issue of meeting nursing home needs is even more urgent for the veteran population than for the general population because the veteran population is older. In 2004, 38 percent of the nation's veteran population was over the age of 65, compared with 12 percent of the general population. Similarly, in Hawaii, 38 percent of the veteran population was over the age of 65, compared with almost 14 percent of the general population.

In my remarks today I will discuss trends in VA's overall nursing home care expenditures,[3] trends in the number of patients served, or "patient workload," and key challenges VA faces in planning for nursing home care for veterans. Examination of data on trends in the provision of nursing

---

[1] In addition to operating expenses, VA also pays about two-thirds of the costs of construction for state veterans' nursing homes.

[2] VA noninstitutional services include home-based primary care, homemaker/home-health aid, adult day health care, skilled home health care, and home-respite care.

[3] These expenditures do not include construction costs.

home care and of challenges VA faces in planning for nursing home care is important for oversight and strategic planning. Examination of these data is also useful in assessing whether the nursing home program is meeting current goals. My comments today are based primarily on work we have previously completed.[4] We updated information from our prior work with spending and patient workload data for fiscal year 2005 that VA provided. Thus we present the most current information available at the time of our November 2004 report[5] alongside the most current information available now to assess trends between these two points in time. For fiscal year 2005, VA used a different cost accounting system to develop expenditure totals for each nursing home setting. VA told us that the accounting system used in fiscal year 2005 would result in higher expenditures than the accounting system VA used in fiscal year 2003. VA could not provide the 2005 expenditure totals using the 2003 cost accounting system, which could be used to determine the extent to which the change in expenditures resulted from real changes in the level of nursing home care expenditures or from the change in cost accounting systems. As in our previous work, we measured patient workload by using the average daily census, which reflects the average number of veterans receiving nursing home care on any given day during the course of the year. In doing our work, we discussed the updated information with VA, determined the information was adequate for our purposes, and incorporated comments from VA as appropriate. We conducted our review from December 2005 through January 2006 in accordance with generally accepted government auditing standards.

In summary, VA's reported overall nursing home care expenditures in its three settings increased from $2.3 billion to almost $3.2 billion from fiscal year 2003 through fiscal year 2005. VA officials attributed the expenditure increase from fiscal year 2003 to fiscal year 2005, in part, to a change in the cost accounting system used to develop expenditure totals for each nursing home setting. Based on VA's reported expenditures, VA-operated nursing homes continued to account for about three-quarters of VA's overall nursing home care expenditures in fiscal year 2005, as they did in fiscal year 2003. In fiscal year 2005, 77 percent of nursing home care expenditures were accounted for by VA-operated nursing homes, compared to 73 percent in 2003. VA spent the remainder on state veterans'

---

[4] See Related GAO Products at the end of this statement.

[5] See GAO, *VA Long-Term Care: Oversight of Nursing Home Program Impeded by Data Gaps*, GAO-05-65 (Washington D.C.: Nov. 10, 2004).

nursing homes and community nursing homes. From fiscal year 2003 through fiscal year 2005, the percentage of overall expenditures for state veterans' nursing homes declined from 15 to 12 percent and the percentage of overall expenditures for community nursing homes declined from 12 to 11 percent.

VA's overall patient workload in nursing homes increased to an average of 34,375 patients per day by fiscal year 2005, 3.5 percent above the fiscal year 2003 workload. State veterans' nursing homes accounted for over half of VA's patient workload in fiscal year 2005. The workload percent is higher than the 12 percent expenditure in state veterans' nursing homes partly because VA pays on average about one-third of the costs for care veterans receive in state veterans' nursing homes, compared to the full cost in other settings. From fiscal year 2003 through fiscal year 2005, the percentage of workload provided in state veterans' nursing homes increased from 50 to 52 percent. In contrast, the percentage of patient workload provided in VA-operated nursing homes declined from 37 to 35 percent. The percentage of workload in community nursing homes stayed the same at 13 percent.

VA faces two key challenges in planning for the provision of nursing home care. The first challenge is estimating who will seek care from VA and what their nursing home care needs will be. This includes estimating the number of veterans that will be eligible for nursing home care, based on law and VA policy, and the extent to which these veterans will be seeking care for short-stay postacute needs or long-stay chronic needs. A second key challenge VA faces is determining whether it will maintain or increase the proportion of nursing home care demand it meets in each of the three nursing home settings or whether veterans will need to rely more on other non-VA nursing home care providers that are funded by other programs, such as Medicaid and Medicare.

Background

VA has provided nursing home care to veterans for over 40 years. The Veterans Millennium Health Care and Benefits Act (Millennium Act)[6] made important changes in VA's nursing home program. This act required that through December 31, 2003, VA provide nursing home care to veterans

---

[6]Pub. L. No. 106-117, §101(a)(1), 113 Stat. 1545, 1547-51 (1999).

with a service-connected disability rating of 70 percent or greater,[7] veterans requiring nursing home care because of a condition related to their service, and veterans who were receiving care in a VA nursing home on November 30, 1999. Subsequent law extended these provisions through December 31, 2008.[8] VA also has established a policy to provide nursing home care to veterans with a 60 percent service-connected disability rating who also were classified as unemployable or permanently and totally disabled. For all other veterans, VA provides care in VA-operated nursing homes and contract community nursing homes on a discretionary basis, depending on available resources, with certain patients having higher priority, including veterans who require postacute care after a hospital stay. VA pays a portion of the cost to treat veterans who seek care in state veterans' nursing homes.

The state veterans' nursing homes receive VA funds as part of their participation in VA's program. As of fiscal year 2005, 116 state veterans' nursing homes in 44 states and Puerto Rico received payment from VA to provide care. In fiscal year 2005, VA paid $59.36 per day per veteran to these state veterans' nursing homes and awarded grants to states for renovations to existing facilities or construction of new state veterans' homes. States are responsible for obtaining financing sources to pay for their portion of veterans' daily cost of care and for their portion related to renovations to existing facilities or construction of new state veterans' homes.

Most veterans, however, do not receive their nursing home care from the VA program but instead receive it from other providers. Care from others includes both long-stay nursing home care to assist with daily activities, such as eating and bathing, and short-stay care requiring skilled nursing home care following hospitalization. For veterans who do not receive their nursing home care from the VA program, care is financed by programs such as Medicaid, Medicare, private health or long-term care insurance, or

---

[7]A service-connected disability is an injury or disease that was incurred or aggravated while on active duty. VA classifies veterans with service-connected disabilities according to the extent of their disability. These classifications are expressed in terms of percentages—for example, the most severely disabled veteran would be classified as having a service-connected disability of 100 percent. Percentages are assigned in increments of 10 percent.

[8]The Veterans Health Care, Capital Asset, and Business Improvement Act of 2003, Pub. L. No. 108-170, § 106 (b), 117 Stat. 2042, 2045-46.

"self-financing" by the patients.[9] States administer Medicaid programs that include coverage for long-stay nursing home care. State Medicaid programs are the primary funders of nursing homes, and self-financing is the next most common source. Medicare primarily covers acute care health costs and therefore limits its nursing home coverage to short stays. Private health insurance pays for a smaller portion of nursing home expenditures than the other three main sources.[10]

Reported Overall Nursing Home Expenditures Increased, with VA-Operated Nursing Homes Continuing to Account for Almost Three-Quarters of Expenditures

VA's reported overall nursing home care expenditures increased from $2.3 billion to almost $3.2 billion from fiscal year 2003 through fiscal year 2005. (See table 1.) Expenditures increased in each nursing home setting. From fiscal year 2003 through fiscal year 2005, expenditures increased by $743 million in VA-operated nursing homes, $80 million in community nursing homes, and $30 million in state veterans' nursing homes. VA officials attributed the expenditure increase from fiscal year 2003 to fiscal year 2005, in part, to a change in the cost accounting system used to develop expenditure totals for each nursing home setting.[11]

---

[9]VA is not authorized, in most cases, to bill and collect payments from Medicaid and Medicare, nor can VA bill other insurers for health care services that are related to a service-connected disability. However, a veteran's eligibility to participate in VA's nursing home program does not prohibit him or her from using these financing sources for nursing home care outside of VA's health care system, if eligible.

[10]See GAO, *Long-Term Care: Aging Baby Boom Generation Will Increase Demand and Burden on Federal and State Budgets*, GAO-02-544T (Washington, D.C.: Mar. 21, 2002).

[11]The change in cost accounting systems may explain why the annual growth in nursing home expenditures from fiscal year 2003 to fiscal year 2005 of over 18 percent was more than double the growth rate of almost 8 percent from fiscal year 1998 through fiscal year 2003.

Table 1: Change in Reported Nursing Home Care Expenditures, Fiscal Years 2003 and 2005

Dollars in millions

Nursing home setting	FY 2003	FY 2005	Change from FY 2003 to FY 2005
VA-operated nursing homes	$1,697	$2,441	$743
Community nursing homes	$272	$352	$80
State veterans' nursing homes	$352	$382	$30
Total	$2,321	$3,174	$853

Source: VA.

Note: Dollar amounts may not add due to rounding. VA officials attributed the increase in expenditures during this period, in part, to a change in the cost accounting system used to estimate expenditures for each nursing home setting.

Based on VA's reported nursing home care expenditures, VA-operated nursing homes continued to account for about three-quarters of VA's overall nursing home care expenditures in fiscal year 2005, as they did in fiscal year 2003. (See fig. 1.) In fiscal year 2005, 77 percent of nursing home care expenditures were accounted for by VA-operated nursing homes, compared to 73 percent in 2003. From fiscal year 2003 to fiscal year 2005, the percentage of overall expenditures for state veterans' nursing homes and community nursing homes declined. The percentage of overall expenditures for state veterans' nursing homes declined during this period because expenditures in VA-operated nursing homes increased more rapidly than expenditures for state veterans' nursing homes. Growth in the percentage of overall nursing home expenditures accounted for by VA-operated nursing homes, as well as the decline in community nursing homes during this 3-year period, was similar to the pattern we observed from fiscal year 1998 through fiscal year 2003.[12] In contrast, the percentage of overall nursing home expenditures accounted for by state veterans' nursing homes increased in the prior period, but decreased from fiscal year 2003 through fiscal year 2005.

---

[12] See GAO-05-65.

Figure 1: Percentage of Reported Overall Nursing Home Care Expenditures by Setting, Fiscal Years 2003 and 2005

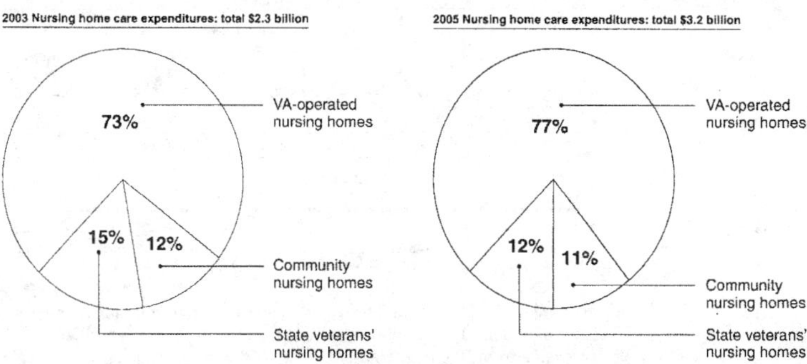

Source GAO analysis of VA data

Note: We calculated these percentages based on VA's reported nursing home care expenditures, which were based on expenditure totals from different cost accounting systems VA used in each fiscal year.

Overall Patient Workload Increased Slightly, with State Veterans' Nursing Homes Continuing to Account for about Half of VA's Overall Patient Workload

VA's overall patient workload in all three nursing home settings, as measured by average daily census, increased to an average of 34,375 patients per day by fiscal year 2005, 3.5 percent above the fiscal year 2003 workload. (See table 2.) However, the small increase in overall workload masked different workload trends in VA's three settings. Strong growth in state veterans' patient workload offset a small increase in community patient workload and a decline in VA-operated patient workload. From fiscal year 2003 through fiscal year 2005, average daily patient workload in the nursing homes VA operated declined by 215, whereas workload in community nursing homes increased by 221 and workload in state veterans' nursing homes increased by 1,155. The continued strong growth in workload in state veterans' nursing homes largely contributed to growth in overall patient workload during this 3-year period and was consistent with the trends that we observed from fiscal year 1998 through fiscal year 2003.

Table 2: Change in Patient Workload, Fiscal Years 2003 and 2005

Average Daily Census

Nursing home setting	FY 2003	FY 2005	Change from FY 2003 to FY 2005
VA-operated nursing homes	12,373	12,158	(215)
Community nursing homes	4,202	4,423	221
State veterans' nursing homes	16,639	17,794	1,155
Total	**33,214**	**34,375**	**1,161**

Source VA.

Note: The workload measure is average daily census, which represents the total number of days of nursing home care provided in a year divided by the number of days in the year.

The percentage of workload provided in state veterans' nursing homes continued to account for about half of VA's overall patient workload, increasing from 50 percent in fiscal year 2003 to 52 percent in fiscal year 2005. In contrast, the percentage of patient workload provided in VA-operated nursing homes declined. The percentage provided in community nursing homes stayed the same. (See fig. 2.) In fiscal year 2005, state veterans' nursing homes accounted for over half of VA's overall workload, and they accounted for 12 percent of overall expenditures for patient care. The relatively low proportion of expenditures can be explained in large part by VA's per-diem rate for care in state veterans' nursing homes, which on average accounts for about one-third of the cost for care in this setting. Continued growth in the percentage of overall patient workload accounted for by state veterans' nursing homes during this 3-year period was similar to the pattern we observed from fiscal year 1998 through fiscal year 2003.

Figure 2: Percentage of Overall Patient Workload by Setting, Fiscal Years 2003 and 2005

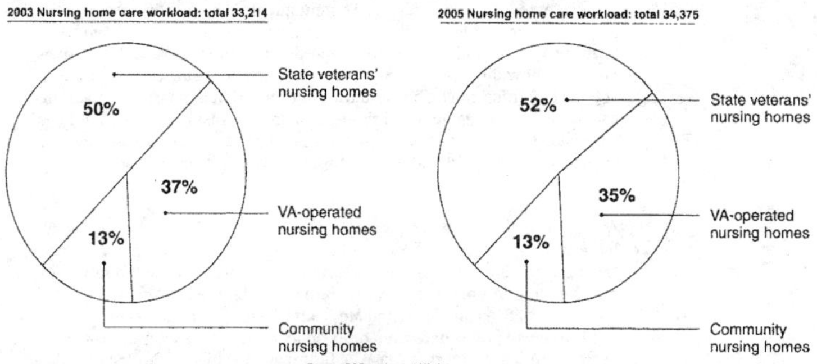

Source: GAO analysis of VA data

Note: The workload measure is average daily census, which represents the total number of days of nursing home care provided in a year divided by the number of days in the year.

VA Faces Two Key Challenges in Planning for Nursing Home Care

VA faces two key challenges in planning for the provision of nursing home care. The first challenge is estimating who will seek care from VA and what their nursing home care needs will be. To do this, VA will need to estimate the number of veterans that will be eligible for nursing home care based on the Millennium Act and VA policy or that will be able to receive such care on a discretionary basis, based on available resources. Moreover, VA will need to estimate the extent to which these veterans will be seeking care for short-stay postacute needs or long-stay chronic needs. To meet this challenge, VA needs to establish a baseline for current nursing home needs being met by obtaining more complete information on the eligibility of veterans currently receiving services and on whether they are using short-stay or long-stay nursing home care. Although VA collects data on eligibility and length of stay for its VA-operated nursing homes, it lacks comparable data on eligibility and length of stay for state veterans' nursing homes and on length of stay for community nursing homes. We recommended in November 2004 that VA work to close this gap.[13] VA agreed to do so, but has not fully implemented our recommendations. VA

---

[13]GAO-05-65.

has begun to collect and report eligibility data on veterans receiving care in VA community nursing homes. Data on eligibility and length of stay for state veterans' nursing homes and community nursing homes are especially critical because these two settings account for almost two-thirds of VA's overall nursing home workload. Without these data, VA does not know how the three settings in combination are being used to serve veterans of different eligibility, and what proportion of short-stay and long-stay needs are being met in all three settings. As a result, VA does not have a baseline from which to estimate future demand for nursing home care in each setting as the overall veteran population and its needs change over time.

A second key challenge VA faces is determining whether it will maintain or increase the proportion of nursing home care demand it meets in each of the three nursing home settings or whether veterans will need to rely more on other non-VA nursing home care providers that are funded by other programs, such as Medicaid and Medicare. To meet this challenge, VA needs to make policy determinations concerning which veterans it will provide nursing home care to in the future and the mix of short-stay and long-stay services it will offer. For example, to what extent will VA continue to provide nursing home care to veterans in addition to those that it is required to serve under the Millennium Act? To what extent will VA provide short-stay nursing home care, and to what extent will it provide long-stay nursing home care? VA told us that such policy decisions have not been made. These policy decisions are needed to establish criteria to be used to identify which veterans VA will serve and what nursing home services it will offer as a matter of policy, in addition to those required by law. Then VA can begin to generate the information it needs for planning. This may include, for example, how many nursing homes are needed in each setting and where they should be located.

VA is working on these challenges and has developed a draft long-term care strategic plan. Completing the long-term care strategic plan could help VA determine how to maximize the use of resources for meeting nursing home needs of veterans across the country in each of the three nursing home settings. VA has not given a timeline for completion of the long-term care strategic plan. In May 2004, the Secretary of Veterans Affairs acknowledged that a strategic plan would be necessary to help achieve VA's goals, including ensuring that veterans have access to an appropriate range of services.[14]

Mr. Chairman, this concludes my prepared remarks. I will be pleased to answer any questions you or other Members of the Committee may have.

Contact and Acknowledgments

For further information, please contact Laurie E. Ekstrand at (202) 512-7101 or ekstrandl@gao.gov. Individuals making key contributions to this testimony include James C. Musselwhite, assistant director, Roseanne Price, and Thomas A. Walke.

[14]Department of Veterans Affairs, Secretary of Veterans Affairs: CARES Decision (Washington, D.C.: May 7, 2004). The Capital Asset Realignment for Enhanced Services (CARES) was designed to assess VA's buildings and land ownership in light of expected demand for VA inpatient and outpatient health care services through fiscal year 2022. Through this process, VA sought to determine what health care services veterans would need in what locations.

Related GAO Products

VA Health Care: Key Challenges to Aligning Capital Assets and Enhancing Veterans' Care. GAO-05-429. Washington D.C.: August 5, 2005.

VA Long-Term Care: Oversight of Nursing Home Program Impeded by Data Gaps. GAO-05-65. Washington, D.C.: November 10, 2004.

VA Long-Term Care: More Accurate Measure of Home-Based Primary Care Workload Is Needed. GAO-04-913. Washington, D.C.: September 8, 2004.

VA Long-Term Care: Changes in Service Delivery Raise Important Questions. GAO-04-425T. Washington, D.C.: January 28, 2004.

VA Long-Term Care: Veterans' Access to Noninstitutional Care Is Limited by Service Gaps and Facility Restrictions. GAO-03-815T. Washington, D.C.: May 22, 2003.

VA Long-Term Care: Service Gaps and Facility Restrictions Limit Veterans' Access to Noninstitutional Care. GAO-03-487. Washington, D.C.: May 9, 2003.

Department of Veterans Affairs: Key Management Challenges in Health and Disability Programs. GAO-03-756T. Washington, D.C.: May 8, 2003.

VA Long-Term Care: The Availability of Noninstitutional Services Is Uneven. GAO-02-652T. Washington, D.C.: April 25, 2002.

VA Long-Term Care: Implementation of Certain Millennium Act Provisions Is Incomplete, and Availability of Noninstitutional Services Is Uneven. GAO-02-510R. Washington, D.C.: March 29, 2002.

VA Long-Term Care: Oversight of Community Nursing Homes Needs Strengthening. GAO-01-768. Washington, D.C.: July 27, 2001.

GAO's Mission	The Government Accountability Office, the audit, evaluation and investigative arm of Congress, exists to support Congress in meeting its constitutional responsibilities and to help improve the performance and accountability of the federal government for the American people. GAO examines the use of public funds; evaluates federal programs and policies; and provides analyses, recommendations, and other assistance to help Congress make informed oversight, policy, and funding decisions. GAO's commitment to good government is reflected in its core values of accountability, integrity, and reliability.
Obtaining Copies of GAO Reports and Testimony	The fastest and easiest way to obtain copies of GAO documents at no cost is through GAO's Web site (www.gao.gov). Each weekday, GAO posts newly released reports, testimony, and correspondence on its Web site. To have GAO e-mail you a list of newly posted products every afternoon, go to www.gao.gov and select "Subscribe to Updates."
Order by Mail or Phone	The first copy of each printed report is free. Additional copies are $2 each. A check or money order should be made out to the Superintendent of Documents. GAO also accepts VISA and Mastercard. Orders for 100 or more copies mailed to a single address are discounted 25 percent. Orders should be sent to: U.S. Government Accountability Office 441 G Street NW, Room LM Washington, D.C. 20548 To order by Phone: Voice: (202) 512-6000 TDD: (202) 512-2537 Fax: (202) 512-6061
To Report Fraud, Waste, and Abuse in Federal Programs	Contact: Web site: www.gao.gov/fraudnet/fraudnet.htm E-mail: fraudnet@gao.gov Automated answering system: (800) 424-5454 or (202) 512-7470
Congressional Relations	Gloria Jarmon, Managing Director, JarmonG@gao.gov (202) 512-4400 U.S. Government Accountability Office, 441 G Street NW, Room 7125 Washington, D.C. 20548
Public Affairs	Paul Anderson, Managing Director, AndersonP1@gao.gov (202) 512-4800 U.S. Government Accountability Office, 441 G Street NW, Room 7149 Washington, D.C. 20548

PREPARED STATEMENT OF THOMAS M. DRISKILL, JR., PRESIDENT AND CHIEF
EXECUTIVE OFFICER HAWAII HEALTH SYSTEMS CORPORATION

Senator Akaka, and other distinguished Members of this Committee, thank you for this opportunity to testify before you in strong support of healthcare programs, services, and facilities that serve the approximately 118,000 Veterans living in Hawaii. Hawaii Health Systems Corporation (HHSC) is grateful for the opportunities to provide high quality healthcare services to Veterans at all 12 of our existing facilities located on five islands of Hawaii. The more than 3,400 employees of Hawaii Health Services Corporation take great pride in caring for our State's Veterans. Soon, our role in caring for Hawaii's Veterans will be expanding to new heights when the 95-bed State Veterans Home is opened for operation and occupancy in 2007.

As Hawaii's Veteran population continues to both grow and age, there is an even more critical need for long-term care services such as will be available in the state-of-the-art State Veterans Home that Hawaii Health Systems Corporation is building in Hilo. This 95-bed facility will significantly increase the number of long-term care (LTC) beds in east Hawaii and because they are earmarked specifically for Veterans and other eligible beneficiaries, we will be measurably improving the LTC access and capacity for our Veterans.

Over the last 8 years, HHSC has enjoyed an outstanding, collaborative and very successful working relationship with the Department of Veterans Affairs-Hawaii, Washington, D.C., the VA Medical & Regional Office Center-Hawaii, the Office of Veterans Services, and multiple Veterans organizations across the State. Since 2001, HHSC has intensively worked with our VA partners to attain the first ever State Veterans Home for Hawaii, and now the fruits of that arduous labor will soon pay off with the opening of the State Home.

We have recently selected and contracted with a nationally acclaimed management company to operate the State Home for HHSC. Community support both in East Hawaii and across the State for our new State Home has been strong and steadfast over the past several years, and we anticipate that this support will continue to grow as we get closer to opening the State Home. The synergy of a combined Federal and State funding of the Home has been the catalyst for making this dream a reality. We deeply appreciate Senator Akaka's tremendous support, as well as the tremendous support we received from Senator Inouye, Representative Abercrombie, Representative Case, Governor Lingle, our Hawaii State legislators, and our Hawaii Veterans organizations in making this State Home possible for Hawaii's Veterans.

We would like to ask for one additional element of support from this Committee and that is to help ensure that the per diem rate for State Veterans Homes is NOT decreased at the Federal level. Decrements to the per diem rate of reimbursement to the State Veterans Home will have serious adverse financial consequences to the viability and sustainability of all State Veterans Home's operations.

Thank you, Senator Akaka, for the tremendous support you continue to give to all of Hawaii's Veterans, and thank you for your sage leadership and the warm Aloha that you bring to our great State.

Mahalo Nui Loa.

PREPARED STATEMENT BY FRANK CRUZ, PRESIDENT KAUAI VETERANS COUNICL
CHAIRMAN FOR THE STATE OFFICE OF VETERANS SERVICE GOVERNORS ADVISORY
BOARD

Chairman Craig, Ranking Member, Senator Akaka, and Members of this Hearing: My name is Frank Cruz. I am a Vietnam Veteran and currently the President of the Kauai Veterans Council and Chairman for the State Office of Veterans Service Governors Advisory Board.

The 95 bed Long Term Care Facility being build in Hilo is a welcome and long awaited project for our veterans living in the State of Hawaii. This Facility will help our veterans especially the World War II, Korean, Vietnam and our 100 percent disabled veterans here in Hawaii a much needed long term care place. However there are some question and information that needs to be decimated to all veterans wanting to apply for this facility.

1. What are the criteria for any veterans applying for long term care?

2. What will be the cost for the veteran and their family?

3. This facility needs professional and trained caretakers, how will this facility be able to be self sufficient without putting the burden on the veterans staying in this facility?

The Kauai Community Based Outpatient Clinic (CBOC) has provided top notch services to our veterans here on Kauai. There are some areas where much needed improvements are needed.

1. Parking for this clinic is inadequate to accommodate for patients having appointment.

2. How will this clinic be able to handle the influx of veterans coming from Iraq and elsewhere?

3. The medical equipment must be up-graded to current standard.

4. There is a need for qualified female to handle the needs for our women coming from Iraq and elsewhere.

5. There is a need to increase manpower and services due to the increased of veteran population returning form the Gulf war.

On behalf of the veterans on Kauai, I thank the members of this Committee for the time you have taken to listen to the concerns of our Island. Your commitment and efforts to our Veteran Community is greatly appreciated. Thank you very much.

PREPARED STATEMENT OF COLETTE V. BROWNE PROFESSOR, UNIVERSITY OF HAWAII SCHOOL OF SOCIAL WORK

Mr. Chairman and Members of the Senate Committee on Veterans Affairs:

Thank you for the opportunity to participate in this hearing on long term care in Hawai'i, and the role of the Department of Veterans Affairs in providing this care.

Mr. Chairman, we at the School of Social Work join in welcoming you to Hawaii. We appreciate your leadership and your commitment to working in a bipartisan manner to better understand how to ensure that the needs of older adults, specifically veterans, are met with accessible and affordable quality of care. I am professor and Chair of the School of Social Work's gerontology program. For more than fifteen years, I have served as a gubernatorial appointment to the State's Policy Advisory Board for Elderly Affairs. In this capacity, I learned a great deal from the older adults in our great State. I also speak to you today as the proud daughter of a World War II veteran. I will speak specifically about the availability of long-term care services in Hawaii.

Long-term care refers to a range of support services provided in a variety of home, community, and institutional settings, and coordinated to meet the needs of people of all ages with disabilities or serious or chronic illnesses. Examples of these services range from personal assistance, transportation, home health, meals, nursing care, case management, and adult day care. Although these services are age-irrelevant, research informs us that the primary consumers are older adults. Nationally, nearly 45 million Americans, or one in every six, are 60 years of age and over. Most older Americans are healthy, contributory members of society. Others, especially those over the age of 85 who compose the fastest growing cohort within the aging population, have become frail and are dependent on others for care. This dramatic shift in our nation's population has clear implications for long-term care, in part because older adults have more chronic ailments than do younger adults. Older citizens account for almost one-quarter of hospital days in 2001, have a higher physician and hospital utilization rate, use 69 percent of home health services, and represent 83 percent of nursing home residents.

Mr. Chairman, Hawaii has one of the Nation's fastest growing aging populations. Today, there are 120,000 citizens who are 60 and over, or 17 percent of our State's population. To put this in perspective, between 1970 and 2000, the older adult population increased by 207 percent while the total population increased by 57 percent. Our life expectancy is greater than any other State—an average of 80 years compared to the Nation as a whole at 77 years. By 2020, an estimated 400,000 residents will be over the age of 60, composing 25 percent of the State's population.

To determine what the State's needs are and may be for long-term care, researchers estimate that 15 percent of citizens have limitations or disabilities that require some form of long term care. In Hawaii, this is estimated to be 31,000 people. It is important to note that of this population, 82 percent have annual incomes of less than $20,000. These are individuals most at-risk of needing public support for long-term care.

Similar to her sister States, Hawaii provides for its disabled and elderly citizens with a wide array of health and supportive care services provided in institutions, health care and social service sites, community based programs and in the home. Over the past twenty years, numerous reports and studies conducted by public and private entities have examined this issue of long term care for Hawaii. A review of these reports finds a great deal of agreement that the long term care system in general is: complex and fragmented, institutionally biased, lacking in its capacity for critical services, limited in its efforts to maximize Federal funding for programs for special needs, supports and services; limited in its agency awareness; and experiencing a shortage of adequately trained professional and direct support workers, especially in rural areas of the State.

Long-term care is not only nursing home beds, although the very frail can be found needing this level of care. According to the Health Care Association of Hawaii, in 2003 Hawaii had fewer than half the national average of long term care beds per 1,000 population aged 65 and over even though we have the fastest growing population in the 85 and over group. The State's nursing facility median occupancy was 93.7 percent. This same report found that Hawai has the most dependent nursing facility residents as measured by higher acuity in areas such as activities of daily living, mobility and medical support requirements. This results in the need for more resources to be utilized in these patients' care. Because of this higher acuity level of Hawaii's nursing facility resident, the average total nursing hours per patient day in Hawaii is 4.57 compared to 3.24 hours per day on the mainland.

To finance existing services, Hawai'i relies on a mix of public and private funders and agencies, together with private and family resources. This is similar to the rest of the nation. Projecting into the future, the Hawaii Health Information Corporation's recent report on forecasting long-term care bed days in Hawaii found that Hawaii's aging population is and will continue to be a challenge for long term care service delivery as baby boomers age. This is because older adults are much more likely to require acute care hospitalization, long-term care, home care and hospice, placing heavy demands on the Medicare and Medicaid programs. This same report found that in both rural and urban settings in Hawaii, the increases in health care utilization are for age related disorders, such as heart disease, diabetes, cancer and stroke. In short, Hawaii 's citizens have the greatest longevity, one of the nation's most rapidly aging populations, the most ethnically diverse population, and, looking at Hawai'i's most frail—the oldest, sickest and most dependent nursing home population in the United States.

Here in Hawaii, the Department of Veterans Affairs (VA) is a key government agency that provides services to veterans on all major islands. Nationally, the Department of Veterans Affairs is responsible for providing Federal benefits to veterans and their families. The most visible of all VA benefits and services is health care, providing a wide spectrum of medical, surgical, and rehabilitative care.

Similar to all public and private agencies, the VA is challenged to meet the needs of this growing population. Unlike other States, Hawaii has two unique characteristics that impact the delivery of care. First, Hawaii's island geography compounds challenges related to access and utilization of services. As an island State, travel must be by plane or boat. Second, our multicultural population is unlike any other State, with a mix of 22 percent Caucasian, 22.8 percent Hawaiian, 11.7 percent Filipino, 16.4 percent Japanese, 16.3 percent mixed, 3.1 percent Chinese, and the category of "other" equal to 7.7 percent. Preferences, cultural values, and practices all influence health status and choice of care. Furthermore, 80 percent of our population resides on the island of Oahu, where most of our main government programs are provided. The State is challenged to ensure that all of its citizens receive equal care. In summary, Hawaii is one of the most ethnically diverse States, has one of the fastest growing aging populations in the nation, and its unique geography lends itself to specific challenges related to access and quality care issues.

As the Nation grows older, Congress is presented with the needs of those who so well have served our nation. In turn, the VA works to meet the needs of its constituencies by responding to recent Congressional laws and mandates within its budgeted resources. This typically results in the prioritization of services. Inpatient rehabilitation, community care, respite services, palliative care and nursing home care are some of the long-term care services offered to veterans through the VA. On our neighbor islands, the VA operates community-based outpatient clinics in their attempts to meet needs. Some services, like homemaker and adult day care, are provided under the Uniform Health benefit to all veterans. Other services, such as nursing home care, are provided under the Millennium Law by contracted community institutions to those with service-connected disabilities.

What we have learned is that veterans and non veterans appear to want the same thing when it comes to long-term care. A recent AARP study found that most adults prefer to receive care in their own home, are not confident about being able to pay for nursing home care; feel it is important for the government to help pay for long term care services, and support being able to decide about the kind of care they want to purchase. It is worth pointing out that it is not only the needs of veterans that must be considered, but those of their families, who have and continue to provide the bulk of long term care. Services to support families, then, must be part of our mix of long-term care.

A critical need in which we at the University see the VA taking a key leadership role is the education and training of new professionals in geriatrics and gerontology. This is no small task, as the recruitment of new professionals continues to be a challenge. The Veterans Administration fulfills a critical and valued community need in its training of future geriatricians, geriatric psychiatrists, and geriatric social workers.

Mr. Chairman, the problems around long-term care are huge, and clearly no one agency can do it alone. Long-term care requires collaboration. Throughout the nation, aging networks, health care providers and community services are joining together to promote and improve the well-being of older adults. A recent report, A Strategic Plan: On Achieving Outcomes on Creating a Legacy: Healthy Aging Project (2005–2009), a partnership among the Aging Network, Department of Health, and public and private agencies here in Hawaii, offered a blueprint for improving health of na kupuna—our elders. This report recommended that any venture to improve the health of our elders must be community driven, inclusive, community-owned, built upon existing community assets and infrastructure to ensure long term sustainability, and use evidence-based strategies. Ensuring the adequacy of the State's infrastructure to provide long-term care requires skilled and knowledgeable professionals and paraprofessionals committed to quality care. From a university perspective, we remain concerned about meeting future long-term care workforce needs. We therefore respectfully request Congressional support for the training and education of future professionals in medicine, nursing, social work and other related fields.

In closing, a recent Summit on Long-Term Care organized by the Hawaii Institute for Public Affairs analyzed previous reports and studies, plans and data, and arrived at the following conclusion. The need exists to build the political will and gain greater community support for the issue of long term care. This hearing can hopefully be seen as a concrete step toward building both.

The VA provides a number of critically important services for our veterans. Nonetheless, they face similar challenges that our State and private entities face: a growing aging population with increasing fiscal restraint. We are all here today because we understand the enormous sacrifice that our soldiers and their families make everyday to serve their country. The question is: Will the Nation be there for our veterans with the necessary long term care services when they need us? The mission of the VA is clear. Have we, in turn, provided them with the requisite resources to meet this need?

I thank you for this opportunity to speak with you today, and I am happy to answer any questions.

PREPARED STATEMENT BY LYNN M. AYLWARD-BINGMAN, CAPT (NC) USNR (RET) MEMBER, VETERANS ADVISORY COUNCIL TO THE VETERANS AFFAIRS PACIFIC ISLANDS HEALTH CARE SYSTEM (VISN 21)

Chairman Craig, Ranking Member, Senator Akaka, and Members of this Hearing: I am Lynn Aylward-Bingman. I am a retired US Navy Nurse Corps Captain. Among other duty stations, I served at the Naval Hospital Guam in 1968—1969 caring for the air-evaced wounded from Viet Nam. Subsequently, while stationed in San Diego, I received my law degree and was a trial attorney for 23 years. I became involved with the Hawaii Veteran community when I came to Kauai, from California, nearly 5 years ago. I am proud to represent our veterans as a member of the Veterans Advisory Council to the VA Pacific Islands Health Care System. In that capacity, my colleagues and I communicate to, and address, concerns of our Hawaii veterans with the Director of the VAPIHCS and the Regional VISN Director. We also liaison with the individual Island Veterans Councils. I am honored to speak on behalf of our veterans, particularly the Kauai veterans, at today's hearing, and to express some of our concerns with the State of veterans' health care in Hawaii.

The citizens of Hawaii are the most patriotic and generous people I've ever known. This is exemplified by the fact that there are several Medal of Honor recipients among our Hawaii veteran community; and by the spirit of "ohana," which is particularly strong in our veteran community. The ohana spirit is very important given the unique disparate and geographic nature of our Islands and the Pacific Region. It is far more difficult for our veterans to obtain full health care services than it is for our fellow veterans on the Mainland.

We are very proud of the strides that have been made by the VA in Hawaii over the last few years, especially those on the Outer Islands such as establishment of Community Based Outpatient Clinics or "CBOCs". Our Kauai CBOC staff are outstanding and do their best to provide a high quality of care to our veteran patient community. However, they are limited in the care they can provide by limited funding. We lack "on Island" VA specialists, certain equipment, and adequate staffing, among other things. There are three areas of concern I would like to address today.

SPECIALIZED TREATMENT/SURGICAL CARE

At present, when a veteran needs specialized care for a cardiac, orthopedic, or serious dermatologic condition, for example, one of three situations will occur after being evaluated by our CBOC staff. The veteran will either: (a) be flown to Honolulu to see a specialist; (b) have to wait several months to get an appointment with one of the specialists who come to the CBOCs intermittently; or (c) obtain authorization to be seen by a local health care provider in the community. Telemedicine greatly assists our CBOC staff in evaluating some health issues, but does not eliminate the need for the veteran to actually be seen and treated by a specialist. Each of the above scenarios costs the VA money and, in the first two, also costs the veteran valuable time.

We recognize that it is not practical, nor possible, to have a full complement of specialists on each Island to see veterans when needed. However, it is also not acceptable to have to wait months, in pain, before a veteran is seen by a specialist who only comes to Kauai for a single day once every 3 or 4 months. Nor is it acceptable to wait several months before the veteran is flown to the Mainland for hip replacement surgery.

When a veteran is flown to the Mainland for surgery, more problems are created. First the VA incurs the transportation costs. Second a sick or disabled veteran is forced to travel alone to a location where he, or she, has no friends nor family support, and undergo, again alone, what is frequently serious or even life threatening surgery or treatment. Following the surgery or treatment, the veteran then travels alone again to return home. He is not followed by his surgeon, nor is his post operative care or recovery monitored, or modified if needed, by anyone who actually did the surgery. This is far from optimal care and, in some instances, would be considered negligent. If post operative problems occur, other healthcare providers, who have no first hand knowledge of the surgery, are involved in the veteran's care. The more providers involved, the greater the chance recovery problems will arise. Additionally, it doesn't make good medical sense, or good care, to expect a person who has just been through major surgery to travel long distances. Just navigating a large airport these days is stressful to a healthy person.

One solution to this problem, and to obviate the VA incurring the costs of the local health care provider on a fee basis, is to increase and implement more long term arrangements with the local healthcare providers on Kauai, and the other Islands. Through the use of Memoranda of Understanding (MOU), or other long term contracts, more veterans could receive care locally, at a reduced cost to the VA. This would also benefit the veteran in that he would not have to leave his home Island, or family, for surgeries. It would also improve the overall quality of the care rendered as the veteran's progress would be monitored by the provider performing the surgery. If adequate facilities exist at Tripler, another alternative is for the VA to hire board certified specialists who can treat and/or perform surgery on veterans as inpatients at Tripler.

Funding for the VA needs to be significantly increased to meet the increased demand for care, not just by our older veterans, but also to ensure that good care is available to our service men and women who are, and will be, returning from the middle East. We also want to ensure that the VA obtains maximum value for the monies budgeted for healthcare. MOUs with local providers will help accomplish this goal.

STAFFING

Interrelated with the above is our concern that the CBOCs have sufficient staff. Adding another physician would allow for more diagnostic evaluations to be done "in house." In turn, some of the fee based costs incurred by the VA for referrals to local providers would be eliminated or, at least, reduced.

At present, we still have a need for at least one more clinic staff, preferably an LVN or person certified to draw blood. The Kauai CBOC does have a part time person who is in the clinic 3 days a week to draw blood, and collect other specimens, which are then sent off Island for processing. Obviously, this creates a delay in getting results, and in treatment when indicated. It also requires a return visit by the veteran if they come on a day the "lab" person isn't there. Emergency laboratory work is done locally on a fee basis. Again, use of an MOU would be useful in reducing the costs to the VA.

The individual who does the tele-medicine support at the CBOC is, inaccurately, "counted" as Kauai CBOC "staff;" but is, in fact, a Honolulu staff person who could be recalled at any time. If any one of the current staff become ill, or are even on vacation, it creates an immediate staff shortage. The Kauai CBOC staff is very devoted to providing optimal care to the veterans they serve, and they do an excellent job. However, insufficient staff translates into delays for patients, and the inability to see more patients.

One problem with determination of staff needs is that an outdated model, based solely on the numbers of patients, is utilized to assess physician, nursing, and support staff needs. Our CNP not only sees patients and assists our physician. She also is responsible for all the patient education, supervision of the staff, dispensing medications, doing follow-up phone evaluations and many other duties. However, the CBOCs needs for additional nursing personnel are based only on the number of patients she sees. All the other hours she expends on the care of our veterans, including preventative care through education, are not counted. The methods used to evaluate the healthcare needs and, hence, determine the amount of funds needed and allocated requires immediate revision and updating.

Of equal import is the long time need for a Home Health nurse. Monies for this position were budgeted and approved; but the monies were utilized for other health care matters. However, the need for a Home Health care nurse still exists. Hawaii, and the Pacific Islands in general, have significant numbers of elderly veterans. Many of these veterans have reached the age when they can no longer drive or tolerate the trip from their homes to the CBOC. The obligation to these aged veterans cannot be ignored or forgotten. Once again the inability to meet these healthcare needs is due to lack of adequate funding to provide these services. Long term care facilities are non existent, but greatly needed, for Kauai veterans. Similarly, Kauai's homeless veterans are in need of attention. Extension of the O'ahu outreach and other programs, even on a part time basis, is needed.

FUNDING

As noted at the outset, VA Pacific Islands Healthcare System encompasses a vast, and disparate, geographic area. The very composition of the System mandates additional monies be allocated for rendering health care, and other, services simply to meet the costs of transportation and the necessity of utilizing community resources more frequently than a similar Mainland veteran population. Our healthcare providers primary goal is to render quality care for our veterans. Although some increases have occurred, the VA budget is still seriously short of it's needs. Providers are doing the best they can, but cannot work miracles . . . with limited staff, resources and equipment, the care rendered is also limited.

On behalf of the veterans we represent, I thank the Members of this Committee for the time you have taken to hold these hearings and listen to the concerns of our Islands. Your efforts and commitment to our Veteran community is greatly appreciated. Mahalo, and Aloha.

PREPARED STATEMENT OF LAURIE MAKANEOLE

I would like to take this opportunity to express my concern regarding our returning military personnel from Iraq and Afghanistan. Kauai will be having over 100 reservists but in addition we have many Kauai people who have also served in the active military and will also be returning from Iraq and Afghanistan.

I have a son who is a Captain out of the Stryker Brigade Combat Team from Fort Lewis-Washington—who just recently returned from Iraq. I am concerned that these military persons and their families need access to Post Traumatic Stress counseling-that is appropriate for them. These young people returning are not the same persons who left us a year ago—and we all need help with this serious issue.

I am concerned about their successful re-entry into our world. These young persons gave so much of themselves and now need our help to assist with a successful re-entry and a good future life. Their difficulties are also a spouse and child concern-it affects the entire family unit.

Please provide funds to appropriately educate families and provide appropriate treatment for this concern.

PREPARED STATEMENT OF MARTIN T. RICE

In the summer of 1966 I joined the U.S. Army and served two tours in Vietnam which just so happened to span three successive Tet Offensives: 1967 and '68 in Nha Trang, on the central coast, and 1969 at Long Binh, just outside of Saigon.

I was told that one of the benefits of joining the service was life-long health care coverage. Some administrations have whittled away at the promise. It is an alarming trend.

However, I am grateful for the partial coverage that has been provided to me. The Government has admitted and taken responsibility for the diabetes and colon cancer that was diagnosed in August of 1999, probably as a result of exposure to Agent Orange during one or both of those two tours. The emphysema that was simultaneously diagnosed in August 1999 is currently not a problem, however, it continues to be monitored and is a result of the cheap tobacco products offered to young soldiers, such as myself, at PX's. I was able to stop smoking, with the help of hypnotherapy, in November 1988, 22 years after entering the service. The emphysema appears to be in check. The diabetes is likewise under control, thanks to the monitoring by Dr. Duvachelle and the Kauai Clinic staff, however, to keep it under control requires the attention and time-frame of a part-time job. I currently spend about 18 hours a week, including drive time, at the gym in order to maintain blood sugar levels. I've found that 6 days a week of cardio-vascular exercise coupled with weight training has done the trick. I am able to forgo medicine, most days, and of course, I watch my diet. I have, over the years, seen the number of per-year visits at the Kauai Cluuc, whittled down, due in part to my exercising regimen, but also due in part to a heavier patient load carried by the staff.

Be that as it may, the lasting effects of the Agent Orange-induced colon cancer are ever-pervasive. I had what's known as a total proctocolonectomy, basically Tripler Army doctors in Honolulu took everything "south" of the small intestine: the appendix, colon and most of the rectum, and reattach the small intestine to what was left of the rectum. The procedure was innovative at the time, and required a 4-month period with a colonectomy bag while the lower third of my small intestine was trained to function, somewhat, as a colon.

I do own my own home-based business, however it requires one day of delivery, from Kekaha to Hanalei—a day of complete fasting until the deliveries are done. Usually that means from the preceding evening until 7pm that day, at the earliest, about 24 hours.

I'm also lucky to have started this business in 1990, as I've been able to adapt it, somewhat, to my current medical condition. Otherwise, I would be unemployable, as the absence of the storage capacity that a colon provides requires many daily restroom visits. By way of measurement, I usually use seven to ten rolls of toilet paper weekly. Literally, I know my way around this island from restroom to restroom.

Additionally, I have not slept more than 4 hours uninterrupted at any given time since the April 2000 surgery, due to the need to use the restroom at all hours, giving rise to what has been diagnosed as acute sleep deprivation.

I'm not complaining. I know many people have it a lot worse than I. I feel lucky to be here, as the cancer surgery, which took place almost 8 months after diagnosis, again due to the heavy patient load, this time at Tripler, came just in time. It became negated as the cancer had spread quite dramatically; a total proctocolonectomy became necessary. It was luckily performed before the cancer penetrated the outer wall of the colon, from which it usually spreads to the liver, a sure death sentence.

I have presented all of the preceding to demonstrate how precarious my current situation is. Without the promise of medical help of the government, I would not have even limited health coverage. In fact, I probably would have been dead already.

I feel that this promise of limited health care is in further jeopardy, for main two reasons. (1) there's a need for increased staffing at the local clinic as the load will be increasing due to returning servicemembers from Iraq and Afghanistan, and (2) there's the ongoing threat that the current administration will cut health services to people such as myself as a matter of fact.

Those who know me, know that I remain active in spite of my service-connected diseases. In addition to my main business and the 6 days-a-week gym workouts, I am starting a second business. I'm also a lobbyist at the State legislature for a civil rights organization, I'm the current chair of the local Democratic Party and I serve as treasurer for a local non-profit.

My story is but one of a hundred thousand in this small State, and one of but millions upon millions nationwide. My dream of public service at the State legislature will probably remain just that, due to the aftermath of my service-connected diseases as I feel that although my country wouldn't abandon me or my health care needs, this Administration will.

PREPARED STATEMENT OF RONALD K. TAKAMURA

Mr. Chairman, Senator Akaka and other distinguished members of the panel. My name is Ronald K. Takamura. I am a medically retired US Army Captain. I am presently involved with the Hawaii Veterans Community and especially on affairs concerning the Veterans of Kauai.

First of all, let me give you a broad insight of just where this island stands within the entire United States. Our little island has a population count of approximately 54,000 people of which approximately 5,700 are veterans; this is equal to 10 percent of the population which is the highest pro-capita ratio in the entire United States. Our CBOC technical staff which consists of only one Doctor, one Nurse Practitioner and one Psychologist see and treat approximately 30+ patients per day out of a registered count of approximately 1,850 veterans. With the returning veterans from the Middle-East who will be coming home very shortly, our facility will be greatly under-staffed and will be very strained to deliver the best care and services to the total number of veterans.

As a proposed remedy to this situation, the following idea is presented to you for your consideration:

A. Facts:

1. The CBOC and the VA office located at its present location will have outgrown its space for which the sum of $ 15,000.00 plus utilities is paid for rent on a monthly basis.

2. There is only adequate parking space for 17 cars including those that belong to the staff.

3. Cost to the VA each time a veteran is sent t Honolulu runs over $200.00 per visit for transportation alone.

4. It takes the veteran approximately 3 hours of travel time to get to Honolulu and another 3 hours for him to return.

5. In addition to the above, the State of Hawaii Office of Veterans' Affairs (OVS) pays approximately $1,850.00 rent for the area it occupies in the present Veterans Center.

B. Proposal:

1. The Kauai Veterans Council has acquired enough additional land at the rear of the present center to construct a two or possibly three story building in which it would be ideal to house the CBOC, VA Office and the OVS Office.

2. This building would be customized to house an expanded CBOC as well as the other offices. By doing so, would create a one-stop Veterans Complex with ample parking and technical facilities to better serve our veterans in the long run.

3. The monies paid for rent/utilities would be better utilized as the facilities located within this complex will be owned by our veterans, and would contribute toward any costs incurred like mortgage, etc.

4. The CBOC would then be expanded to handle a larger technical staff as well as up-to-date equipment and programs which would be classified a State-of-the-Art.

5. The cost of flying specialists to Kauai from Oahu would be cheaper than flying patients from Kauai to Oahu due to the following accepted procedures presently in effect:

a. Time saved on patient travel time which would be an equivalent to approximately 3 hours to and from Oahu for a total of 6 hours.

b. Each time a patient goes there to Oahu, he is first interviewed by interns from the University. The interns then consult with the specialist and only after all of this, he gets to see the specialist for approximately fifteen minutes if lucky. If the specialist flew over to Kauai, there would be no interns and then he would be able to service at least three to four times as many veterans for the same amount of time.

c. Transportation for patients would be much simpler with the utilization of the DAV Transportation Network and the Kauai Bus services.

d. By increasing the technical staff of the CBOC, i.e. one Doctor, one Laboratory Technician, one administrative clerk and one records management clerk, much better services could be provided the veterans and the waiting periods between appointments would be greatly reduced.

As for my comments on Long-Term Care Facilities, I personally do not think that the operation of one on this island would be economically practical. In addition, to have the facility on another island would not for practical purposes sufficiently or efficiently service our veterans due to travel and other cost restrictions.

The cost factors to operate such a facility have not been spelled out to the veterans in black and white which leaves many loop holes in the true benefits that a veteran would gain over the civilian type of care facilities now in operation.

For example, if the administration would only accept the VA benefits check, the Social Security check and maybe $\frac{1}{2}$ of the retired military pay check, then the veteran may be able to benefit some provided that his personal property not be touched. If his personal property and assets are included into the cost factor, then

I contend that there would be no different than the present operating Long-Term Care Centers presently in operation and the veteran would lose in the long run.

Judging from the panel members in attendance of his hearing, all of the operational bodies would belong to a profit making organization or company and would be out there to make money instead of trying to do what would be best for the veteran. Therefore, I contend that there would be better ways to utilize our monies, such as building a center as proposed above.

Thank you for giving me this opportunity of testifying before this Committee.

PREPARED STATEMENT OF WILLIAM T. HONJIXO

A hearing as this is great appreciated by veterans on this island of Kauai. IT certainly demonstrates that our nation cares about veterans. The caliber of participants and speakers were outstanding and impressive. It was not "eye wash," but a serious attempt to solve problems facing the veterans here on Kauai and the State of Hawaii. Mahalo for your effort and the caring of veterans.

○